A2Z inER

A₂Z ᴵᴺ ER

The Clinical Guide in the Emergency Room

Bone fractures – special edition

First edition
2019

Mina Azer

M.B.B.Ch, Master of Surgery

First edition: 2019

First Printing: November 2019

ISBN-13: 9781706918516
Imprint: Independently published

The cover has been designed using resources from rawpixel.com / Freepik

Mina Azer, MSc., MBBCh.

Master of Surgery, Mans. Uni.
Department of general surgery and emergency medicine, Ubbo-Emmius Klinik GmbH.
Oster Str. 110, 26506 Norden, Germany.
Email: meena_tharwat@yahoo.co.uk

ACKNOWLEDGMENT

This work is inspired by my colleagues, both junior and senior. I was lucky enough throughout my career so far to encounter enthusiastic persons who were both eager to learn as well as pass their experience to others. This continuous process of sharing and learning was a main part of my work routine in the Gastroenterology surgical center in Mansoura University and The Egyptian Liver Institute.

I would also like to thank my colleagues in the surgery department in the Ubbo-Emmius Klinik in Norden, Germany, for being really supportive throughout the process of writing this book. I would like to thank Ibram Botros for his valuable insights and Samuel Gendy for his much appreciated technical support. Last but not least, I would like to thank Dr. Hripsime Rüstemyan and Dr. Hans-Uwe Volkers from whom I have learnt a great deal in the last three years.

This work could have never been done without the sincere support and understanding of my brave wife Mariam and my sweet angel Clara. I admit being an annoying person when consumed by a new idea. The good news is, I am done now!

TABLE OF CONTENTS

This book is the second part of A₂ZᵢₙER© series which aims at providing a quick yet comprehensive source for medical care providers in emergency situations.

The beginning of the first night shift ever, is always a scary moment for everyone. The more experienced colleagues are already at home, and probably asleep. You are sitting in the ER or the ED waiting for the next patient, asking yourself, what would it be? A 2 cm cut wound or a perforated appendix? A mild gastroenteritis after an unfortunate fast food meal or a massive myocardial infarction? Knowing that all the possibilities are already lurking in the night outside, makes you a little bit nervous.

A₂ZᵢₙER© is the guide of the junior resident during their lonely night shifts. We assume that you have a good grasp of the basic medical knowledge. So, we won't discuss any theoretical aspects, mechanisms of action, or any other boring topics. All clutter has been ripped down leaving the very core of the addressed topics, bearing in mind the old – but still true – idiom; "common is common". In this book, you will find only the most common answers to the most common questions asked by younger colleagues.

The main idea of these books is to give you a handy tool that I wish I had during my first shifts. A concise guide to what to do and how to do it when you have no one to ask and no time to go through commercials, blocked content and false web search results to find a simple answer.

This is a special edition of A₂ZᵢₙER© the clinical guide in the emergency room focusing on bone fractures. It includes skeletal radiological anatomy with tips and tricks on where to look for a fracture. The second chapter is an illustrated gallery of common bone fractures with commonly used classifications and management options. The third chapter is a new addition to this special edition. It deals with the AO classification basic concepts with a quick user manual and useful algorithms.

My last words to you: know the night philosophy! These could be summarized in the following points:

✓   Your main aim in the ER is not to miss a catastrophe more than to diagnose a rare condition.

✓   Stay focused on the patient's main problem. Do not get lost in the sideways.

✓   Learn to prioritize your actions, deal first with the problem that most likely would kill or deeply harm the patient.

✓ Do not perform any maneuver (diagnostic or therapeutic) during the night shift that could be postponed to the normal working hours in the next morning without harming your patient.

At last, my best wishes to my colleagues all over the world holding their position at night, guarding the human frontier against pain, suffering and death.

Mina Azer

Norden, 09ᵗʰ November 2019

CHAPTER 1: SKELETAL X-RAYS

GENERAL CONCEPTS IN EVALUATING SKELETAL X-RAYS

To evaluate any skeletal x-ray, you must check first its quality. There are three main questions that you should always ask before beginning your evaluation.

I.   Is the data accurate?

    Is this the right patient? The right date? And the right side to be investigated?

II.   Does everything visible?

    There are standard requirements of every x-ray in which a minimum of structures should be visible to evaluate it thoroughly. For example, a long bone x-ray should always include at least one joint in the view. Another example, the hand x-ray. All fingers and the wrist joint should be clearly visible. Don't accept an x-ray with technical failures like an earing blocking the view of a part of cervical vertebrae or a missing little toe in a foot x-ray.

III.   Does everything correctly align?

    Malrotation can dramatically hinder the ability to spot a fracture or a dislocation. Also, malrotation affect all measurement of distances and angles of x-rays rendering these valuable tools useless.

Features of bony fractures seen in plain x-ray.

I.   Primary features

    a.   Gapping and dislocation: presence of a gap in a bony shaft with or without dislocation is the most obvious feature of a fracture.

    b.   Cortical interruption: this is also a very reliable feature of a fracture. It advised to check every cortex of every visible bone on an x-ray film to exclude fractures. Non-dislocated or impacted fractures may present with only cortical interruption.

II.   Secondary features

        a.   Asymmetry: in comparison with the other side.

        b.   abnormal position: loss of alignment or shifting from the normal axis.

        c.   periosteal response: haziness of the area around the fracture due to periosteal effusion.

        d.   trabecular interruption: very prominent feature in fractures of the neck of the femur.

        e.   changes versus old images: especially useful in judging x-rays of older patients suffering from severe degenerative disorders or in patient with old fractures with a suspicious refracture.

In the next pages you will find the most common x-rays encountered in the emergency room setting. For each region you will see a diagram showing the basic radiological anatomy followed by the most common sites of fractures and a systematic way to judge this x-ray.

PELVIS

RADIOLOGICAL ANATOMY

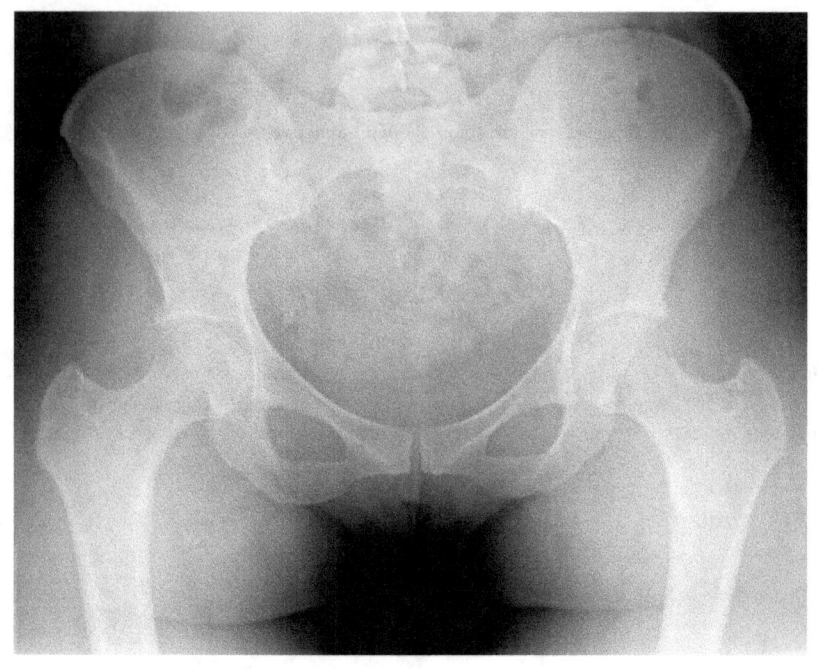

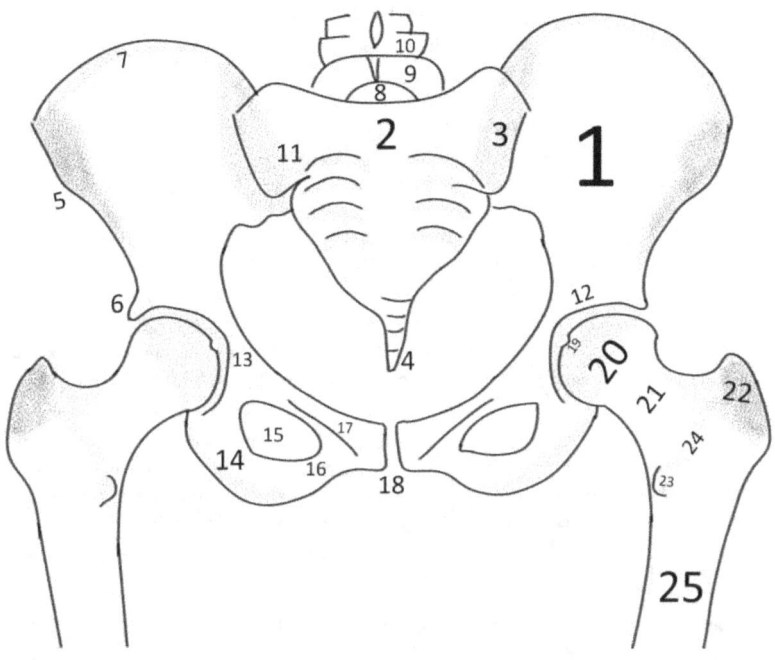

1.	Ileum	15.	Obturator foramen
2.	Sacrum	16.	Inferior pubic ramus
3.	Sacroiliac joint	17.	Superior pubic ramus
4.	Coccyx	18.	Symphysis pubis
5.	Anterior superior iliac spine	19.	Fovea
6.	Anterior inferior iliac spine	20.	Head of Femur
7.	Iliac crest	21.	Neck of femur
8.	Lumbo-sacral joint	22.	Greater trochanter
9.	5th lumbar vertebra	23.	Lesser trochanter
10.	4th lumbar vertebra	24.	Intertrochanteric ridge
11.	Sacral ala	25.	Femur shaft
12.	Acetabulum		
13.	Ischial spine		
14.	Ischial tuberosity		

Pelvic fracture	1	Trace the continuity of the pelvic ring and the obturator foramen for signs of pelvic fractures. Superior and inferior pubic rami are common sites of anterior pelvic fractures.
	2	Confirm the normal appearance of the sacroiliac joint which is a common site of posterior pelvic fractures.
	3	Check the acetabulum for fractures.
Fracture of the neck of the femur	4	Check the neck of femur, greater and lesser trochanter for proximal femur fractures. Look for cortical as well as trabecular interruption.
	5	Shenton's line: any deformity of this line may indicate a fractur of the neck of the femur. This is a imaginary line passing through the inferior border of the superior pubic ramus and the medial side of the neck of femur. normal contour of this line doesn't exclude a fracture.
Avulsion fractures	6	Check the anterior superior/inferior iliac spines for avulsion fractures.

Shenton's line:

In other words; don't trust a normal Shenton's line. It is only a good positive. Deformed Shenton's line without apparent fracture indicates a subtle fracture. That is it!

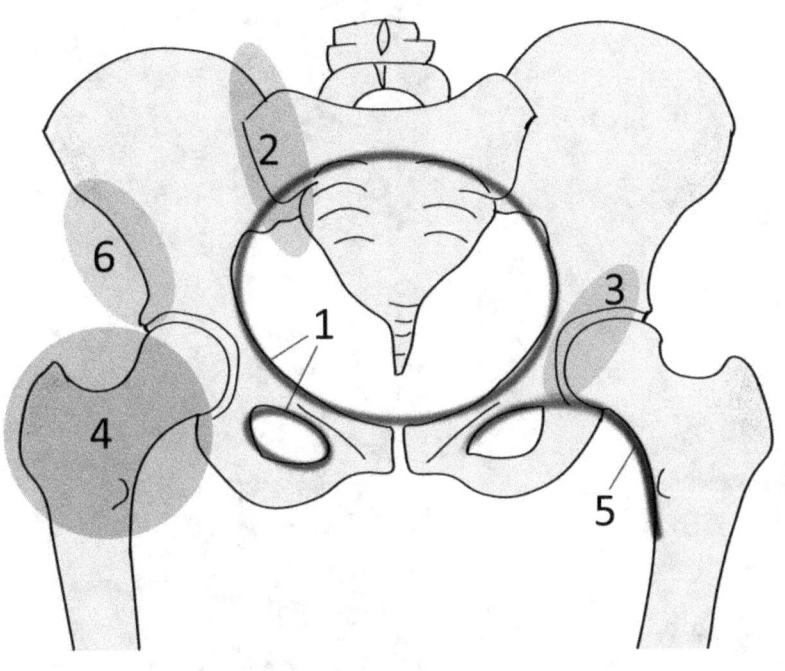

KNEE JOINT

RADIOLOGICAL ANATOMY

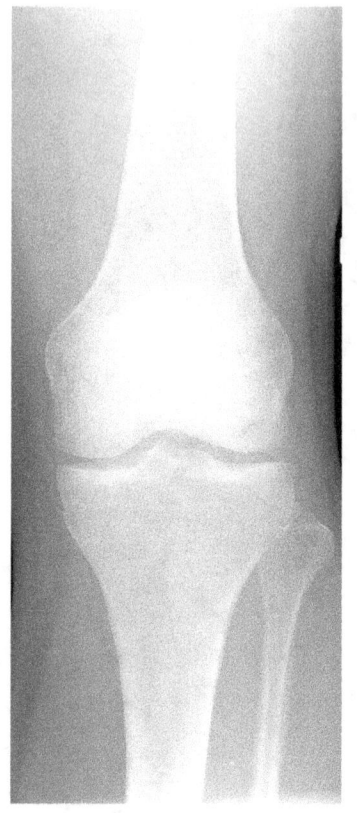 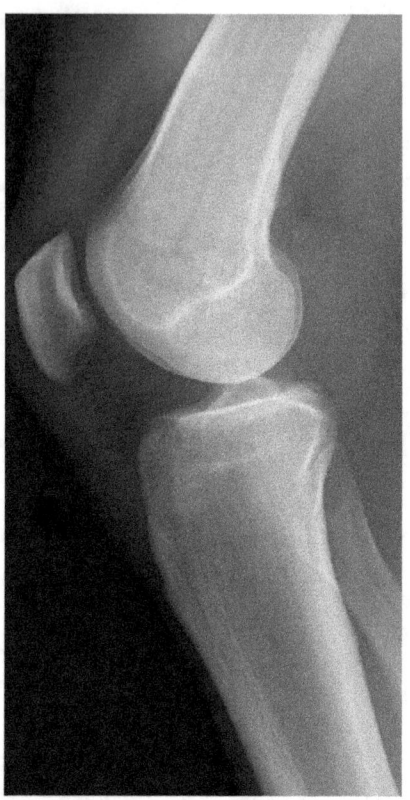

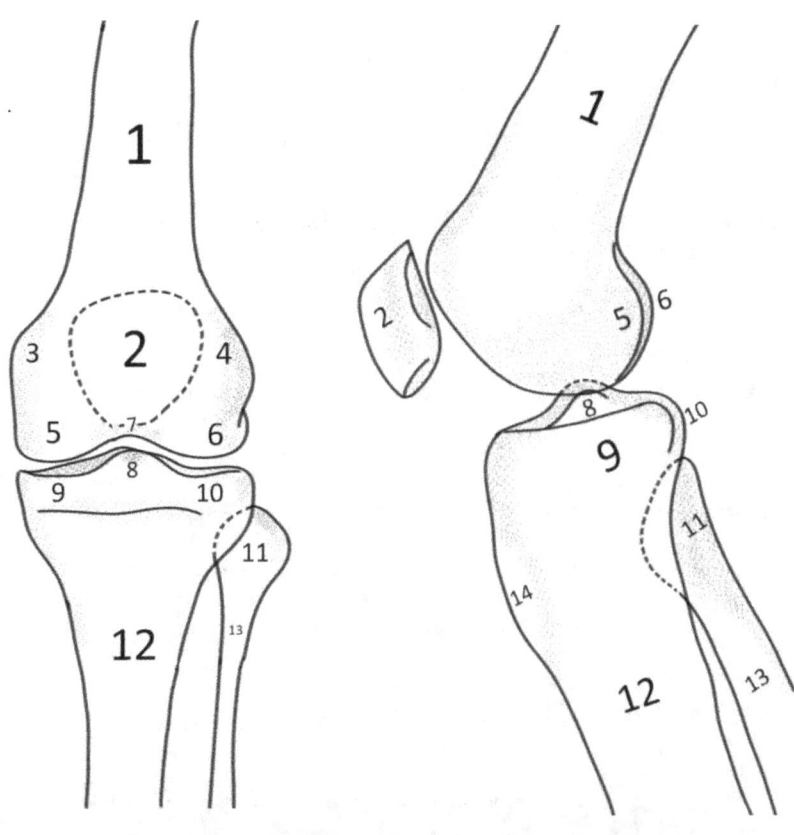

1.	Femur	8.	Intercondylar eminence
2.	Patella	9.	Medial tibial condyle
3.	Medial epicondyle	10.	Lateral tibial condyle
4.	Lateral epicondyle	11.	Head of fibula
5.	Medial femur condyle	12.	Tibia
6.	Lateral femur condyle	13.	Fibula
7.	Intercondylar notch	14.	Tibial tuberosity

Femur fracture	1	Check for supracondylar fracture.
Tibia fracture	2	Check for lateral and medial fracture.
Fibula fracture	3	Check for Maisonneuve fracture specially associated with ankle injury.
Patella dislocation	4	Confirm the normal position of patellar shadow to exclude patellar lateral dislocation.
Normal findings	5	A small sesamoid bone (Famella) may be present in this area.
Soft tissue injury	6	This a common site for seeing a hematoma. The clear distinction between blood and fatty tissue called the FBI sign (Fat-Blood Interface).
Cruciate ligament injury	7	The extension of an imaginary line extending between the roof the intercondylar notch of the femur (a) and the Intercondylar eminence (b) should be always parallel to the posterior cortex of the tibia (c). inclination of this line indicates deviation of the longitudinal axis of the knee joint due to a possible cruciate ligament injury. MRI is the diagnostic test.
Quadriceps or patellar tendon rupture.	8	A bony fragment in this area may indicate an avulsion fracture of the quadriceps tendon.
	9	The direction of patellar dislocation in patellar tendon rupture.
	10	The direction of patellar dislocation in quadriceps tendon rupture.
	11	Blumensaat line is the line drawn along the roof of the intercondylar notch of the femur as seen on lateral radiograph of the knee joint. It can been used for indicating the relative position of the patella as normally this line intersects the lower pole of the patella.
	12	To asses patellar deviation compare the area of contact between the patella and femur (d) and the perpendicular distance between the lower pole of the patella (e) and the flat surface of the tibia. A ratio more the one indicates patellar dislocation.

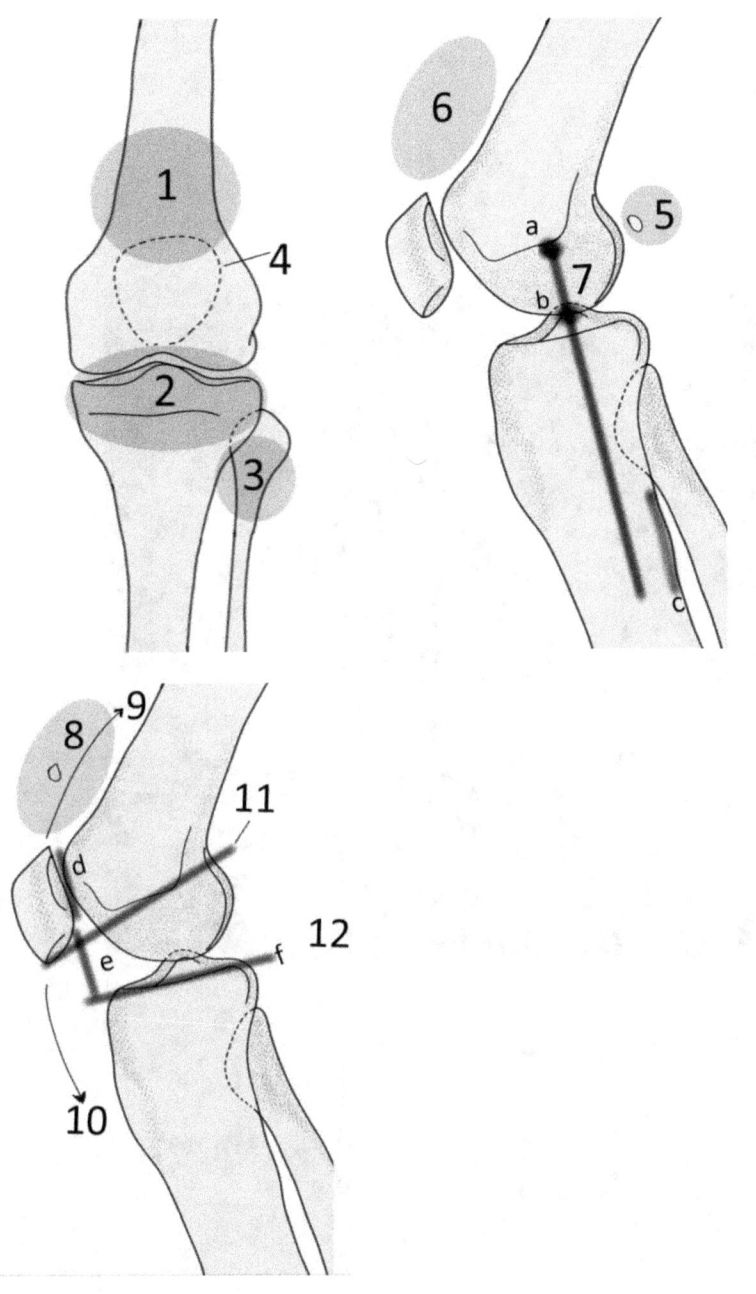

ANKLE JOINT

RADIOLOGICAL ANATOMY

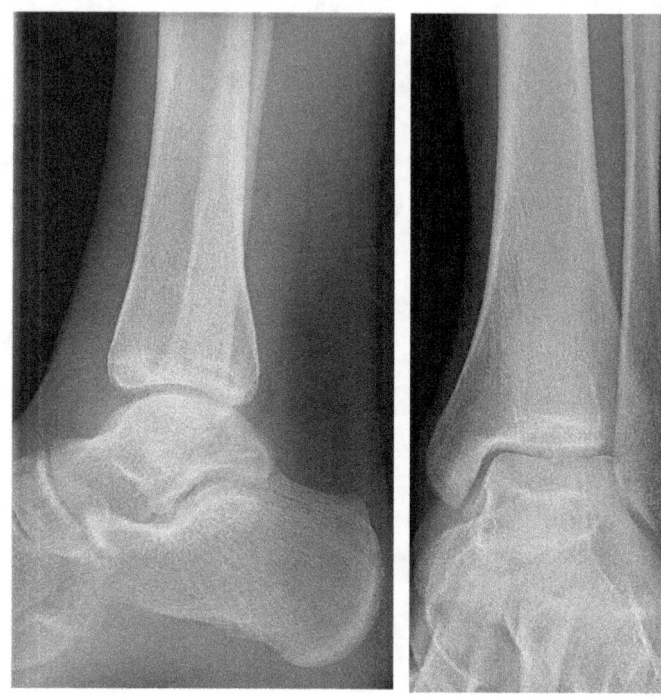

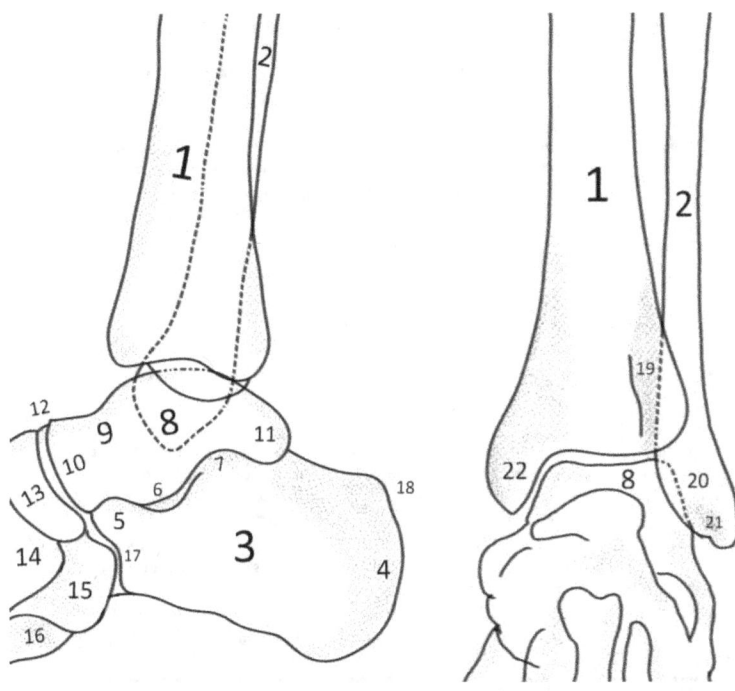

1.	Tibia	12.	Talonavicular joint
2.	Fibula	13.	Navicular
3.	Calcaneus	14.	Medial cuneiform
4.	Calcaneal tuberosity	15.	Cuboid
5.	Anterior process	16.	Base of the 5th metatarsal
6.	Sinus tarsi	17.	Calcaneocuboid joint
7.	Talocalcaneal joint	18.	Achilles tendon insertion
8.	Talus body	19.	Fibular notch
9.	Talus neck	20.	Lateral malleolus
10.	Talus head	21.	Malleolar fossa
11.	Posterior process	22.	Medial malleolus

Lateral malleolus fracture	1	Check for a fracture and its level in comparison with the syndesmoses.
Medial malleolus fracture	2	Check for a medial malleolar fracture sometimes associated with a lateral malleolar fracture. Also look in this area for avulsion fracture associated with deltoid ligament injury.
Syndesmotic injury	3	Check the width of the tibiofibular overlap area (a). This should be measured 1 cm above the tibial plafond. Normally it should be more than 6 mm in anteroposterior images. A smaller area of overlap indicates a widened tibiofibular space, which by turn is an indicator of a syndesmotic injury.
	4	A uniform tibiotalar joint space that measures 3 to 4 mm indicates an intact syndesmosis.
Posterior malleolus fracture	5	Check a fracture at the Volkmann's triangle specially in association of a bimalleolar fracture.
Calcaneal fracture	6	Bohler's angle: is the angle between the anterior and the posterior plane of the calcaneus. The anterior plane is represented by a line between the top of the anterior process (d) and the dome of the calcaneus (c), while the posterior plane is represented by a line drawn between the superior end of the calcaneal tuberosity (b) and the dome of the calcaneus (c). This angle is normally between 20° and 40°. A deviation from these values is an evidence of calcaneal fracture.

> **Normal values:**
> width of the tibiofibular overlap: > 6 mm
> tibiotalar joint space: 3-4 mm
> Bohler's angle: 20°-40°

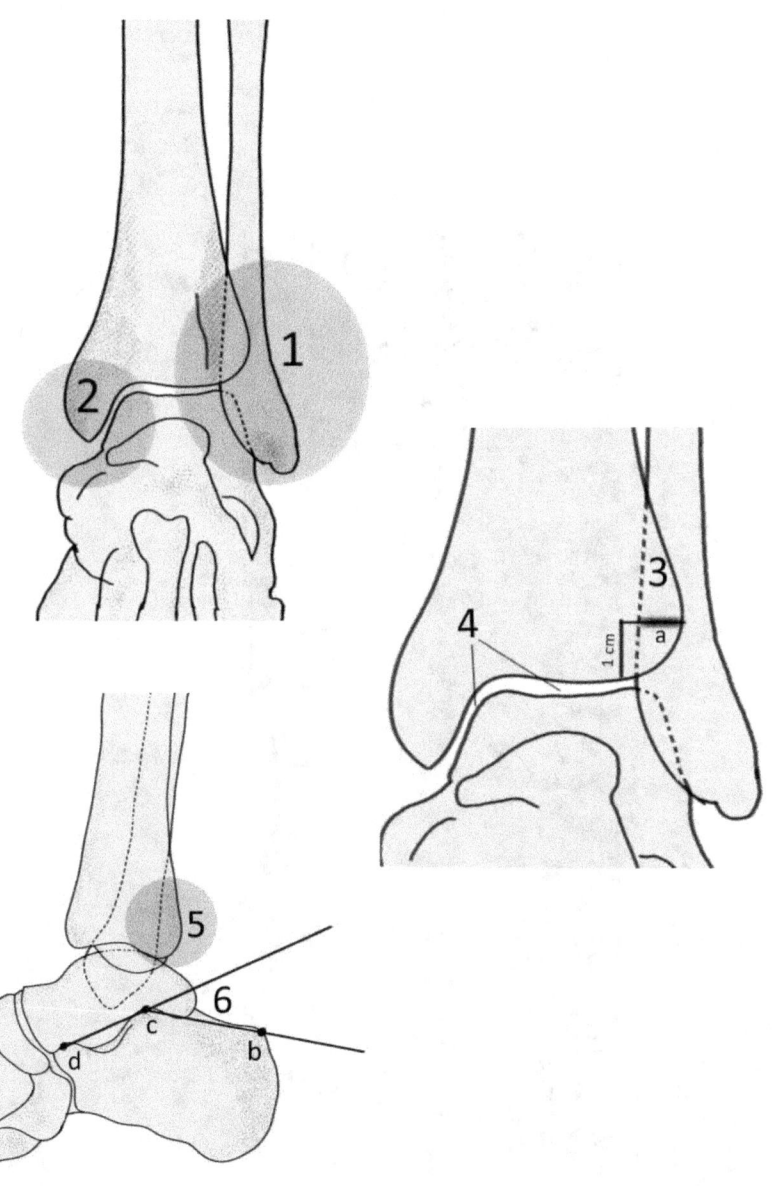

Foot

Radiological anatomy

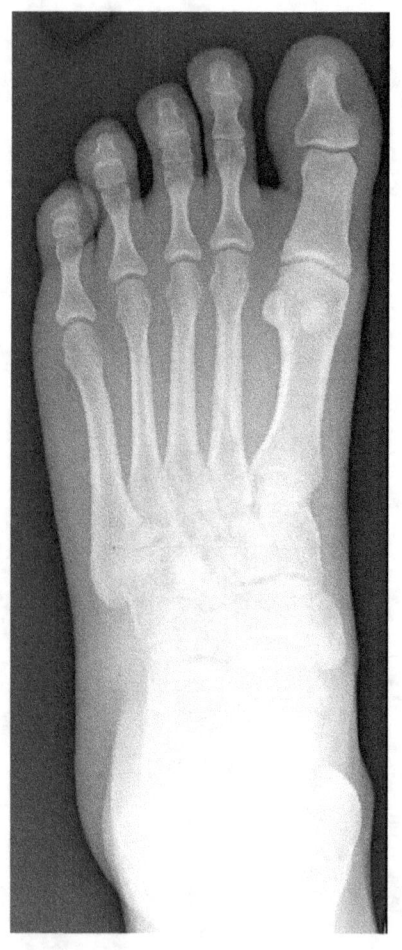

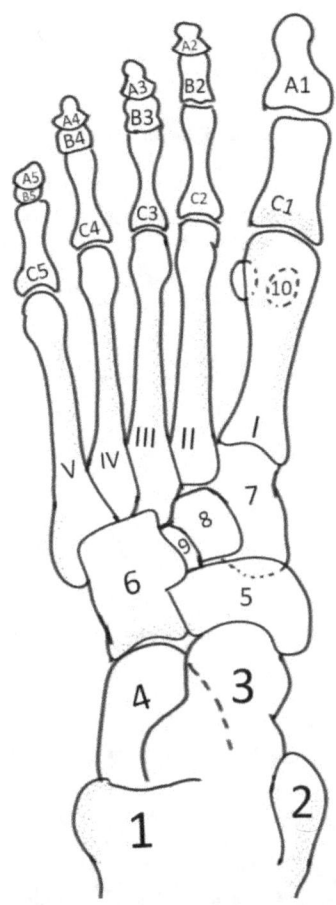

1. Tibia	10. Sesamoid bone
2. Fibula	A1-A5. Distal phalanges
3. Talus	B2-B5. Intermediate phalanges
4. Calcaneum	C1-C5. Proximal phalanges
5. Navicular	I-V. 1st to 5th metatarsals
6. Cuboid	
7. Medial cuneiform	
8. Intermediate cuneiform	
9. Lateral cuneiform	

INTERPRETITION

Proximal 5th metatarsal fracture	1	The most common foot fracture, associated with ankle joint sprain.
5th Toe proximal phalanx and distal 5th metatarsal fracture	2	A common site for dislocation fracture.
Big toe	3	Both phalanges are site of fracture caused by direct trauma.
Proximal 2nd to 4th metatarsal fractures	4	Caused by exaggerated plantarflexion.

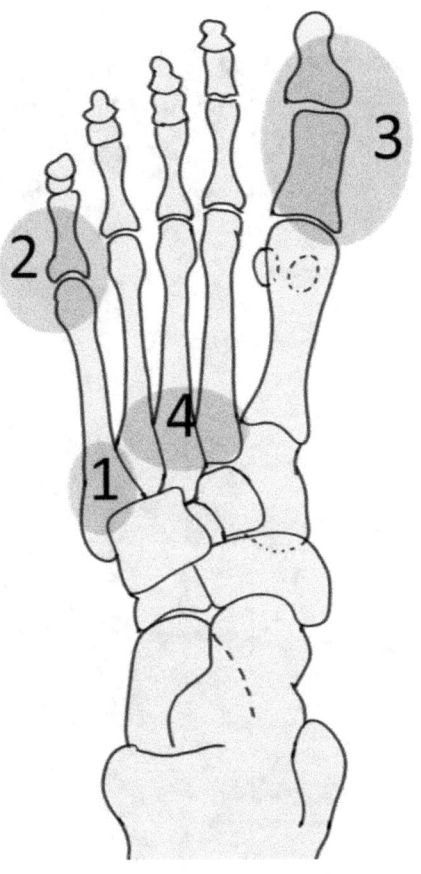

SHOULDER JOINT

RADIOLOGICAL ANATOMY

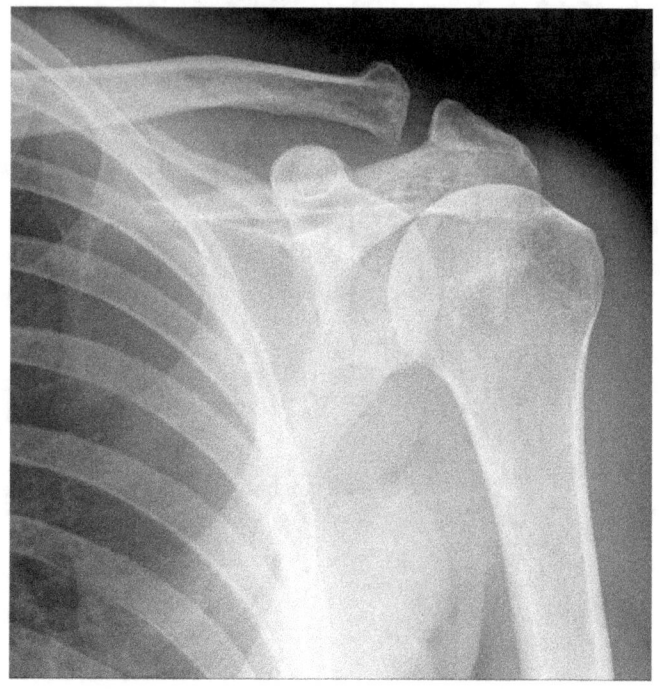

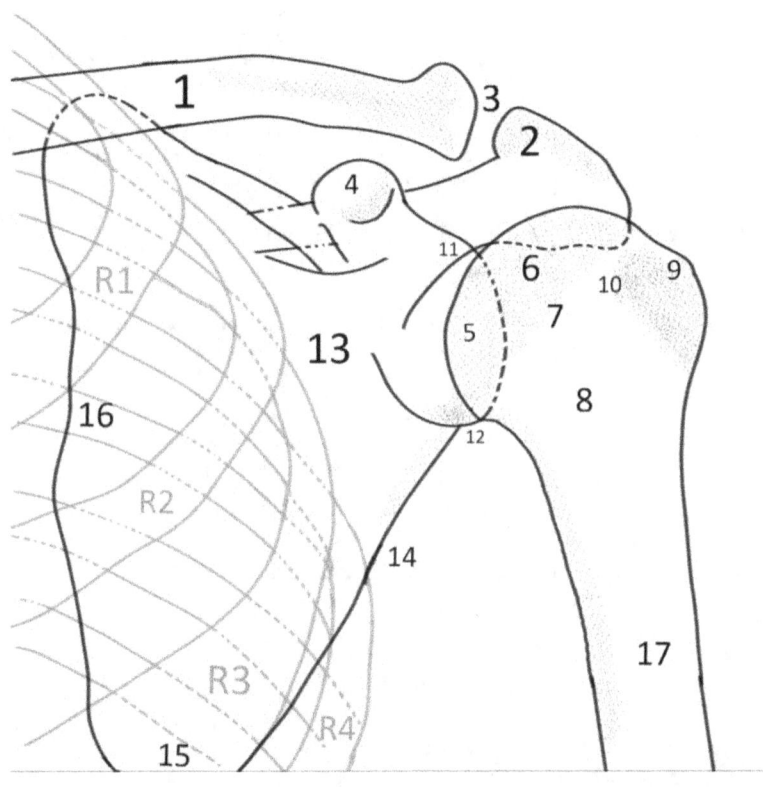

1.	Clavicle	10.	Lesser tuberosity
2.	Acromion process	11.	Supraglenoid tubercle
3.	Acromioclavicular joint	12.	Infraglenoid tubercle
4.	Coracoid process	13.	Scapula
5.	Glenoid cavity	14.	Lateral border of scapula
6.	Head of the humerus	15.	Inferior angle
7.	Anatomical neck	16.	Medial border of scapula
8.	Surgical neck	17.	Shaft of the humerus
9.	Greater tuberosity	R1 – R4. Anterior rips 1 to 4	

Clavicular fracture	1	Look here for a clavicular fracture. This is a common fracture. The proximal fragment is normally superiorly dislocated by the pulling action of the sternomastoid muscle, while the distal fragment is inferiorly dislocated as it is pulled down by the weight of the arm.
Acromioclavicular joint dislocation	2	Asses the level of the clavicle in relation to the acromion. An elevated clavicular lateral end indicates an Acromioclavicular joint dislocation.
Humerus neck fracture	3	Check the proximal humerus for a fracture at the anatomical neck (b) or more common at the surgical neck (a).
Shoulder dislocation	4	Abnormal position of the head of the humerus indicates a dislocation. More than 90% of dislocation are anterior dislocation. It is important to check for an accompanying fracture before trying a reposition. The distance between a head of the humerus and the acromion (c) is normally between 7 and 11 mm. a wider distance indicates a dislocation.
Greater tuberosity avulsion fracture	5	Check this area for an avulsion of the greater tuberosity,

Normal values:
Acromio-humeral distance: 7-11 mm.

✓ Greater distance (> 11 mm) indicates a shoulder dislocation.

✓ Smaller distance (< 7 mm) indicates a rotator cuff injury (mostly chronic injury).

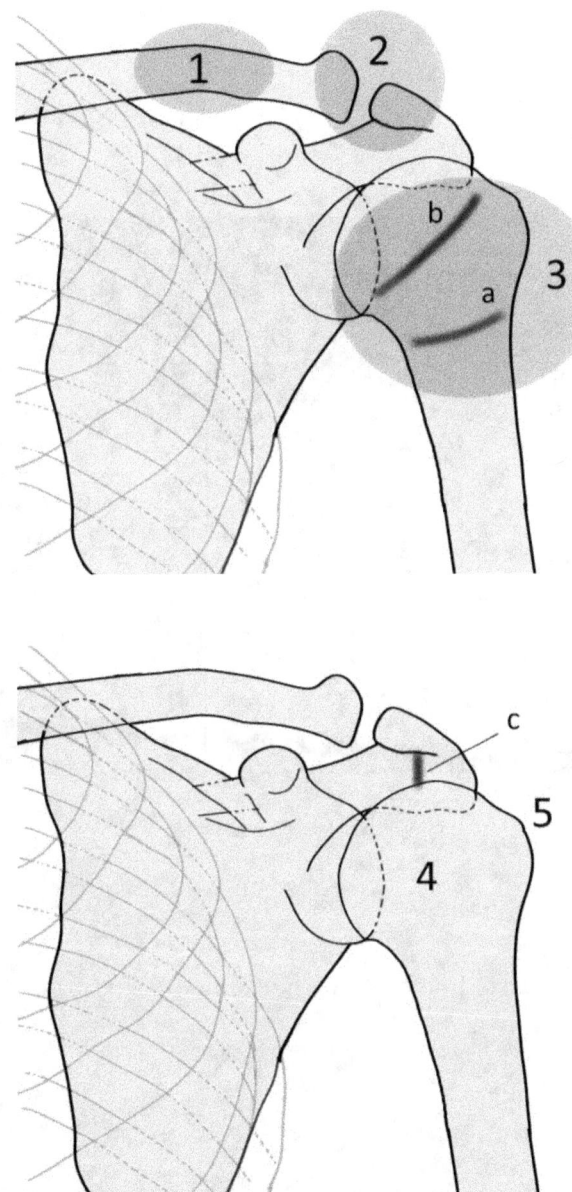

Elbow joint

Radiological anatomy

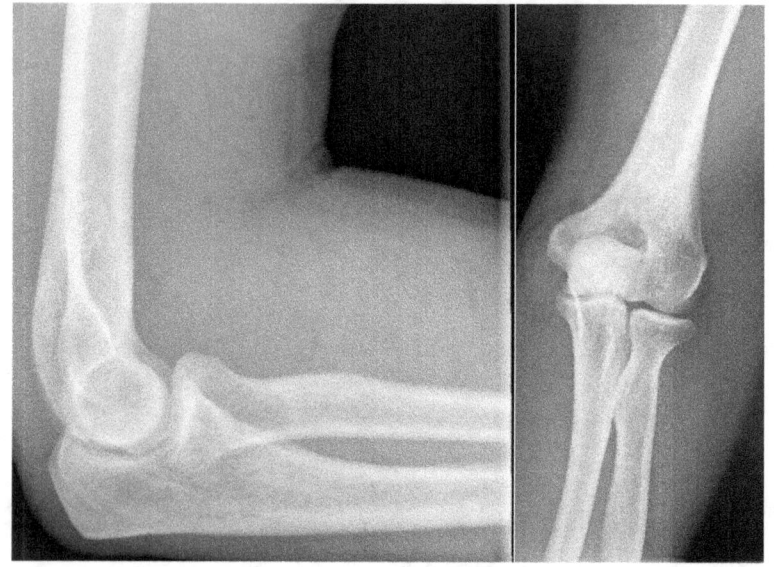

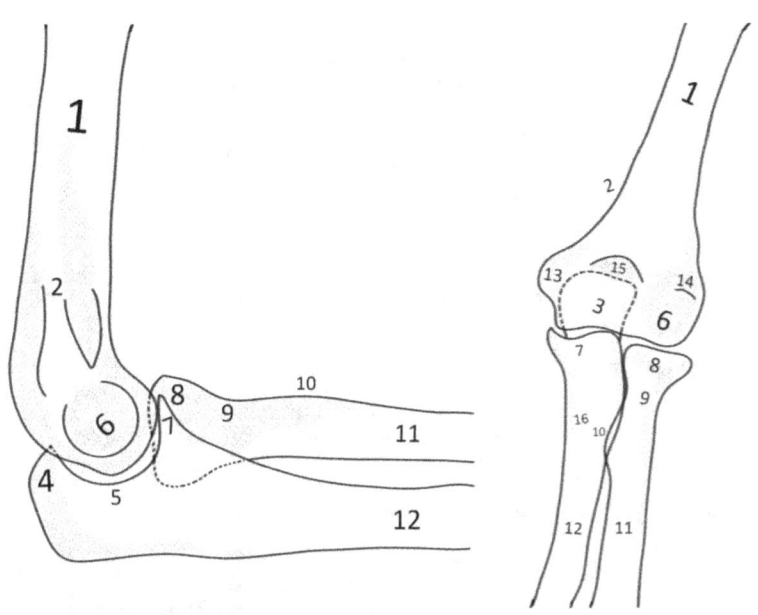

1. Humerus shaft
2. Supracondylar ridge
3. Trochlea
4. Olecranon process
5. Trochlear notch
6. Capitulum
7. Coronoid process
8. Head of radius
9. Neck of radius
10. Radial tuberosity
11. Radius shaft
12. Ulnar shaft
13. Medial epicondyle
14. Lateral epicondyle
15. Olecranon fossa
16. Ulnar tuberosity

Alignment	1	Correct alignment is crucial to judge other aspects of elbow x-ray. This is determined by the presence of a clear figure of "8" formed by the cortical marking of the supracondylar ridge and the capitulum.
Indirect sings of fractures	2	Visible pad of fat could indicate joint effusion caused by a fracture. The pad of fat appears as a darker area (radiolucent) surrounded by normally lighter (radiopaque) soft tissue. Anterior pad of fat (a) could be normally found as a thin shadow. Pathological enlarged anterior pad of fat is called: Sail sign. Posterior pad of fat is always pathological.
	3	Anterior humerus line: passes along the anterior border of the distal humerus. It should always intersect the central part of the capitulum (c). Otherwise is an indication of a dislocation or a fracture.
	4	Radio-capitellar line: passes through the central part of proximal radial shaft. It should always intersect the capitulum and the anterior humerus line at the center of the capitulum (c). Otherwise is an indication of a dislocation or a fracture.
Proximal ulnar fracture	5	The olecranon process is the most common site of ulnar fracture.
Proximal radial fracture	6	Don't miss a fracture at the radius head. It could either clearly visible specially at the articular surface, or barely visible as a kink or slight abnormal angulation at or just above the neck of the radius (d).
Distal humeral fracture	7	A supracondylar humeral fracture is relatively common in children.

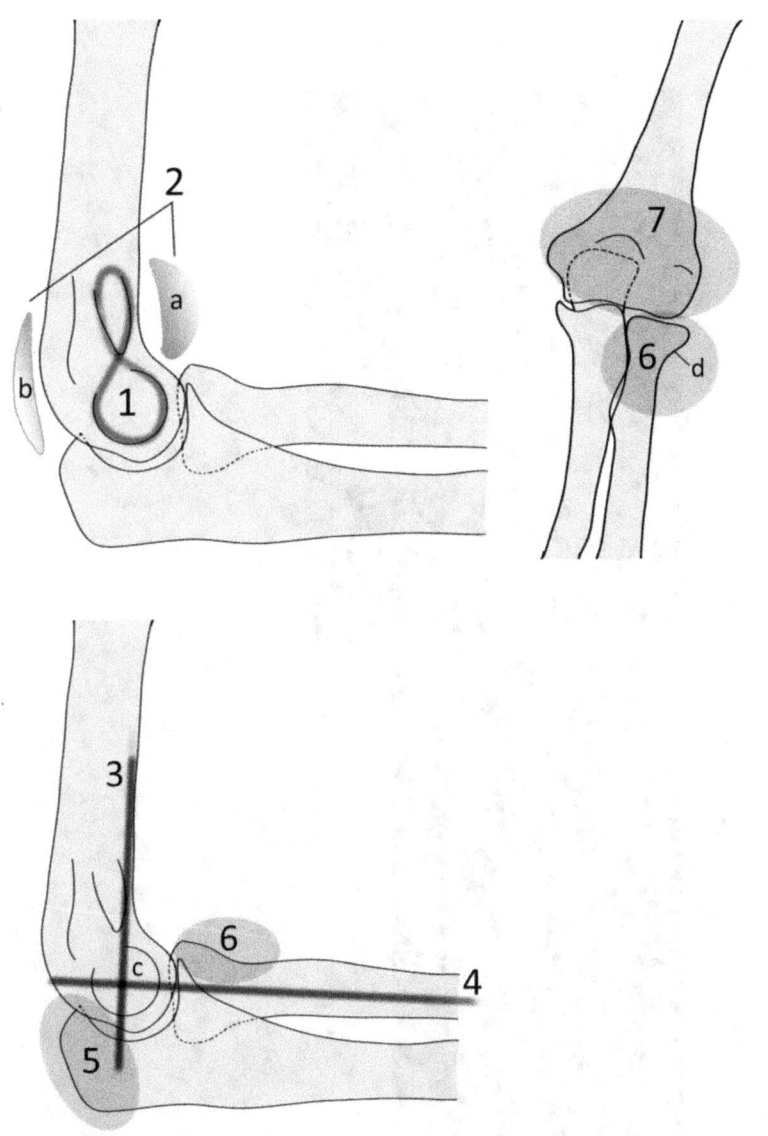

WRIST JOINT AND HAND

RADIOLOGICAL ANATOMY

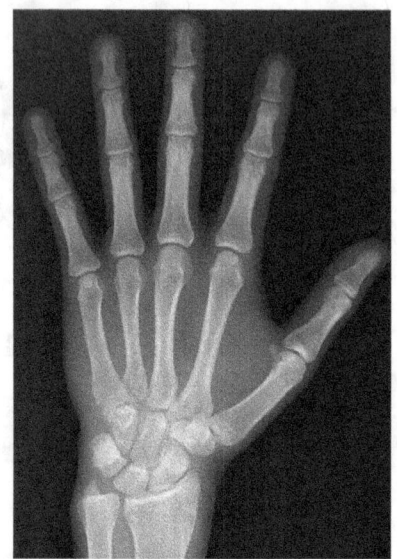

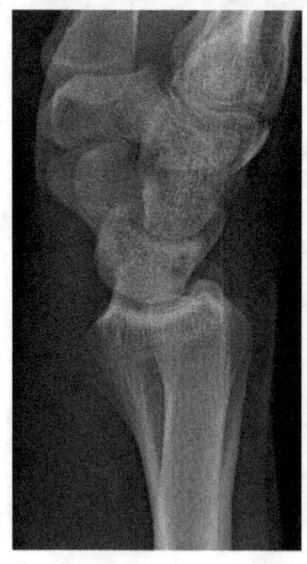

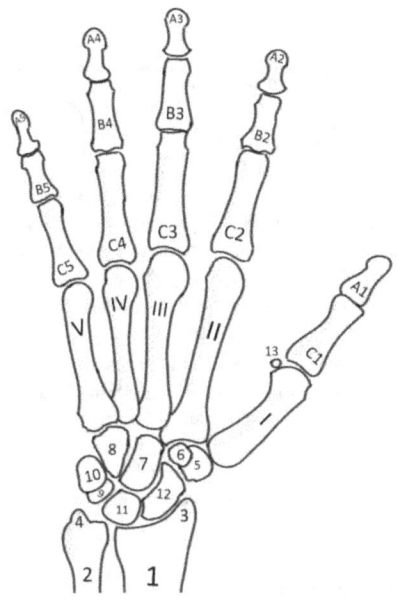

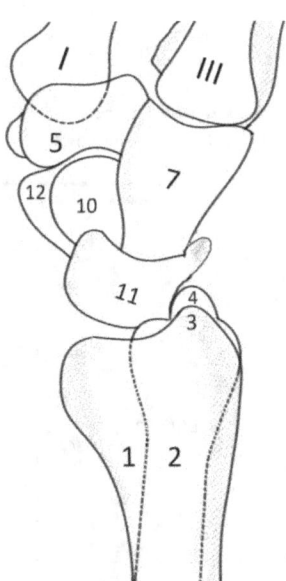

1. Radius
2. Ulna
3. Styloid process (radius)
4. Styloid process (ulna)
5. Trapezium
6. Trapezoid
7. Capitate
8. Hamate
9. Triquetrum

10. Pisiform
11. Lunate
12. Scaphoid
13. Sesamoid bone
A1-A5. Distal phalanges
B2-B5. Intermediate phalanges
C1-C5. Proximal phalanges
I-V. 1st to 5th metacarpals

Metacarpal fractures	1	Boxer's fracture of the head of the 5th metacarpal.
	2	Fracture of the base of the 5th metacarpal.
	3	Rolando's fracture of the base of the 1st metacarpal.
Carpal fracture	4	Scaphoid fracture.
	5	Check the alignment of the capitate, lunate and the radius bone. Malalignment indicates either a perilunate dislocation (only the capitate is dislocated) or a lunate dislocation (only the lunate is dislocated).
	6	a bony fragment in this area indicates a possible triquetral avulsion fracture.
Radial and ulnar fractures	7	Check the contour of the radius for possible fractures
	8	Radial inclination: is the angle between a horizontal plane (a) perpendicular on the radial longitudinal axis (x) and a line drawn between the styloid process and the ulnar corner of the radius (b). normal value is 23°. Smaller angles are called radial tilt that indicates a fracture.
	9	Ulnar variance: is the longitudinal distance between a line tangential to the ulnar articular surface (c) and radius articular surface at the lunate fossa (a). Normal values are between 0 and 2 mm.
	10	Volar and dorsal tilt: is the angle between a horizontal plane (a) perpendicular on the radial longitudinal axis (x) and a line drawn between the styloid process and the ulnar corner of the radius (b). normal value is 11° volar tilt. Further inclination in the direction (d) is a pathological volar tilt. Inclination in the direction (e) is a dorsal tilt which is always pathological.

Normal values:
Radial inclination: 23°
Ulnar variance: 0-2 mm
Volar tilt: 11°
Dorsal tilt: -

AAOS guidelines of operative management*
✓ Radial shortening > 3mm
✓ Ulnar variance > 2mm
✓ Dorsal tilt > 10°
✓ Intra-articular displacement

* American Association of Orthopedic Surgeons

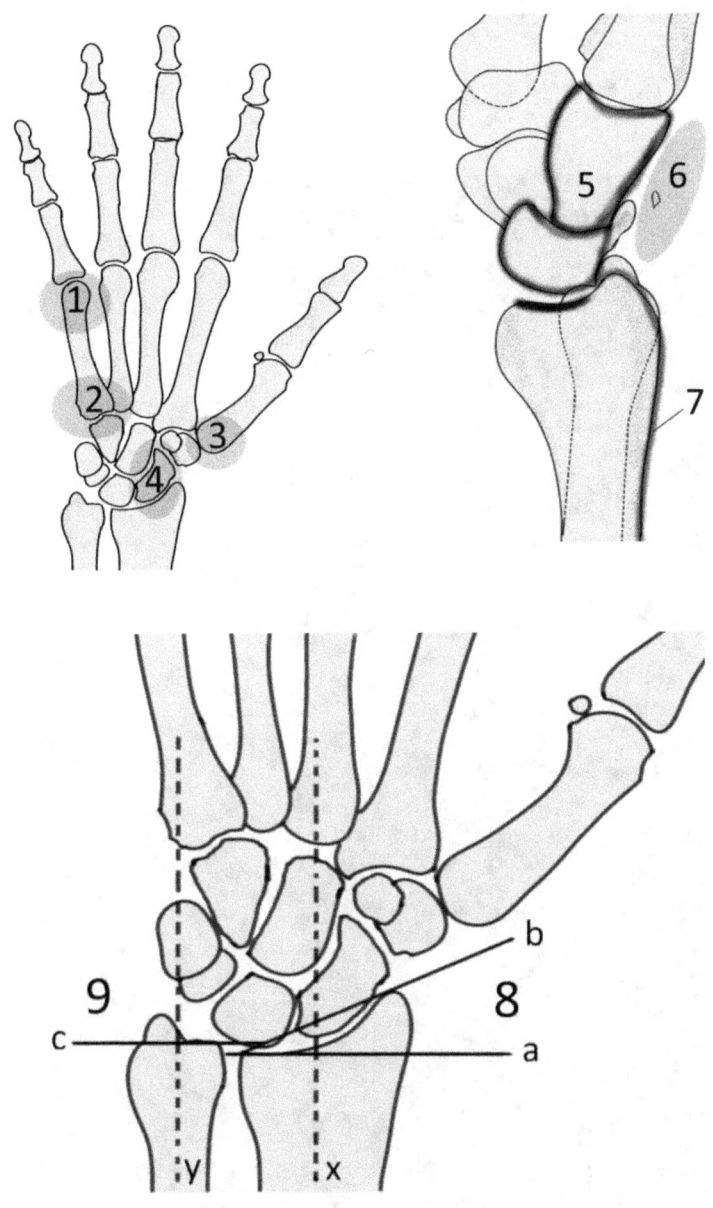

LUMBAR VERTEBRAE

RADIOLOGICAL ANATOMY

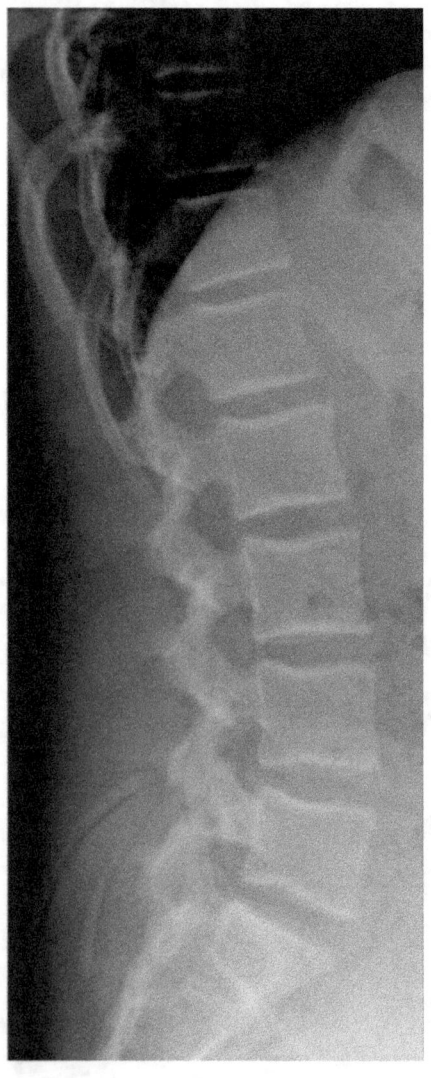

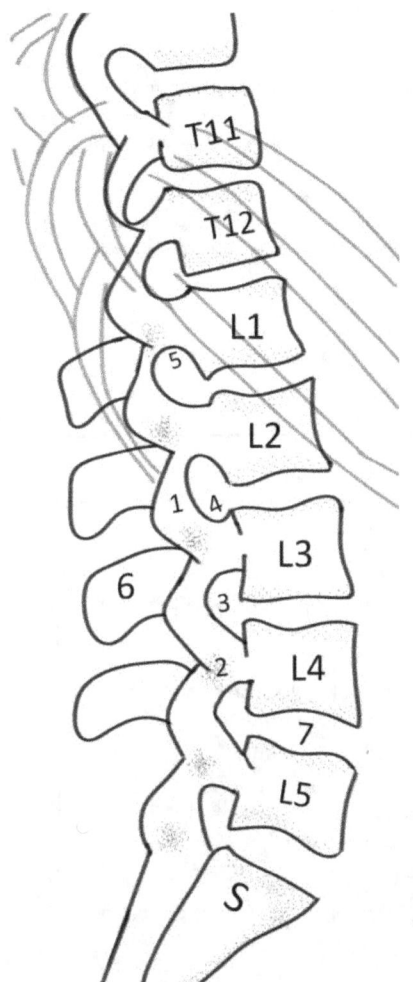

1. Inferior articular process
2. Pedicle
3. Intervertebral foramen
4. Inferior vertebral notch
5. Superior vertebral notch
6. Spinous process
7. Intervertebral desc space
T11-12. thoracic vertebra
L1 – L5. lumbar vertebrae
S. Sacrum

Leveling	1	Identify the 12th thoracic vertebra by the attachment of the last rip.
		Identify the last lumbar vertebra (5th or 6th) which is just above the sacrum.
		In 25% of the population a Lumbosacral transitional vertebra could be identified. It is an extra vertebra that could be considered to belong to sacral (sacralized L5 segment) or lumbar vertebrae (lumbarised S1 segment).
Alignment	2	Check the alignment of all visible vertebrae for dislocated or protruding vertebrae. Loss of alignment could be an indication of a fracture.
Vertebral height	3	Loss of height is an indication of a fracture.

3 common types of vertebral fractures

✓ Compression fracture: only loss of height without loss of alignment.

✓ Burst fracture: loss of both height and alignment (due to anterior protrusion of the fractured vertebra)

✓ Chance fracture: a horizontal fracture of the 3 columns of the vertebra with possible gaping of the spinal processes posteriorly.

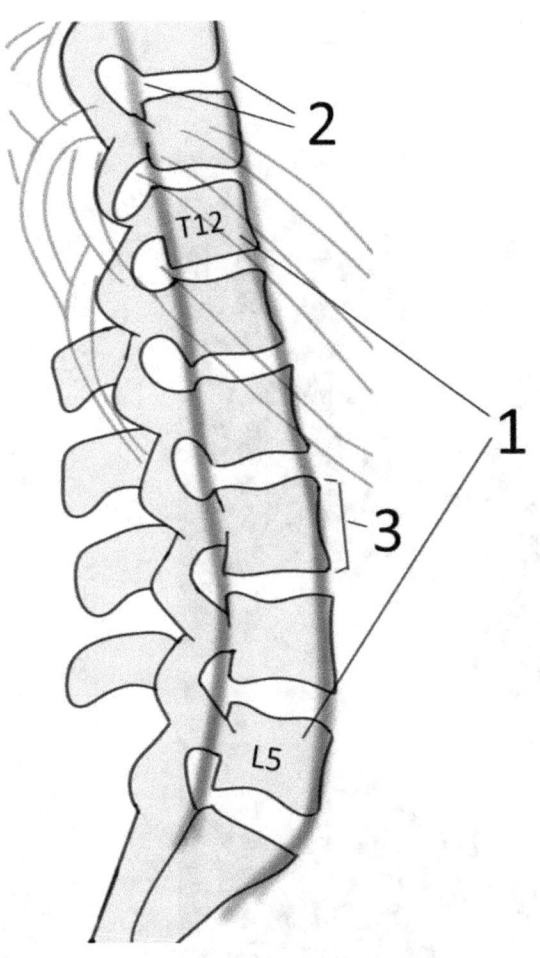

T12

2

1

3

L5

CERVICAL VERTEBRAE

RADIOLOGICAL ANATOMY

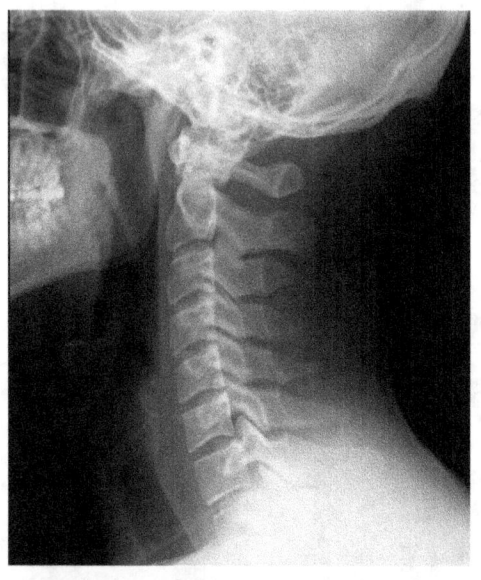

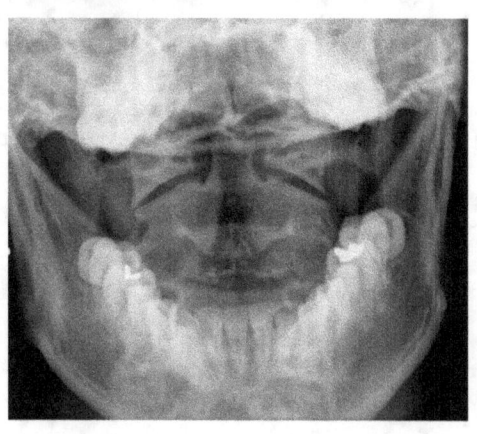

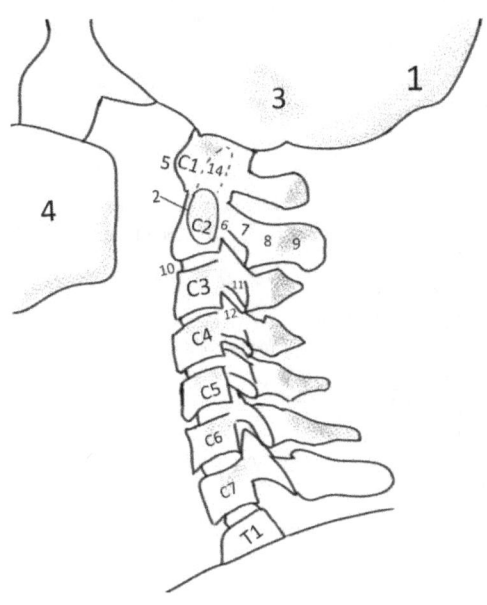

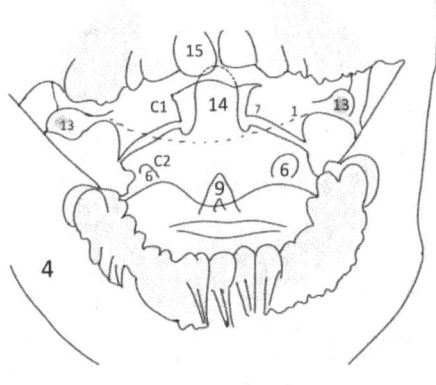

1.	Occiput
2.	Harris ring
3.	Mastoid air cells
4.	Mandible
5.	Anterior arch of C1
6.	Pedicle
7.	Lateral mass
8.	Lamina
9.	Spinous process
10.	Intervertebral desc space
11.	Superior facet
12.	Inferior facet
13.	Transverse process C1
14.	Odontoid process
15.	Central incisors
C1 – C7. Cervical vertebrae	
T1. 1st thoracic vertebra	

Leveling	1	Determine the level of C1 and T1. Both should be visible in an adequate cervical x-ray.
Alignment	2	Check the alignment of the cervical vertebrae for signs of dislocation or fractures through observing 3 longitudinal lines: (a) The anterior line formed by the anterior longitudinal ligament. (b) The posterior line formed by the posterior longitudinal ligament. (c) The spinolaminar line formed by the anterior edges of the spinous processes. Note that the spinal cord (x) lies between the posterior line and the spinolaminar line.
Vertebral height	3	Loss of height is an indication of a fracture. Note that this rule doesn't apply to C1 which lack a vertebral body.
Odontoid process fracture	4	Disruption or a step seen in the cortical ring at the level of C2 is an indicator of odontoid process fracture. This ring is formed the lateral masses of C2 viewed from the side. It is also known as Harris ring.
	5	Look for a visible fracture of the odontoid process.
	6	Lateral process should be aligned in the same plane.
	7	The spaces between the lateral masses of C1 and the odontoid process should be equal.

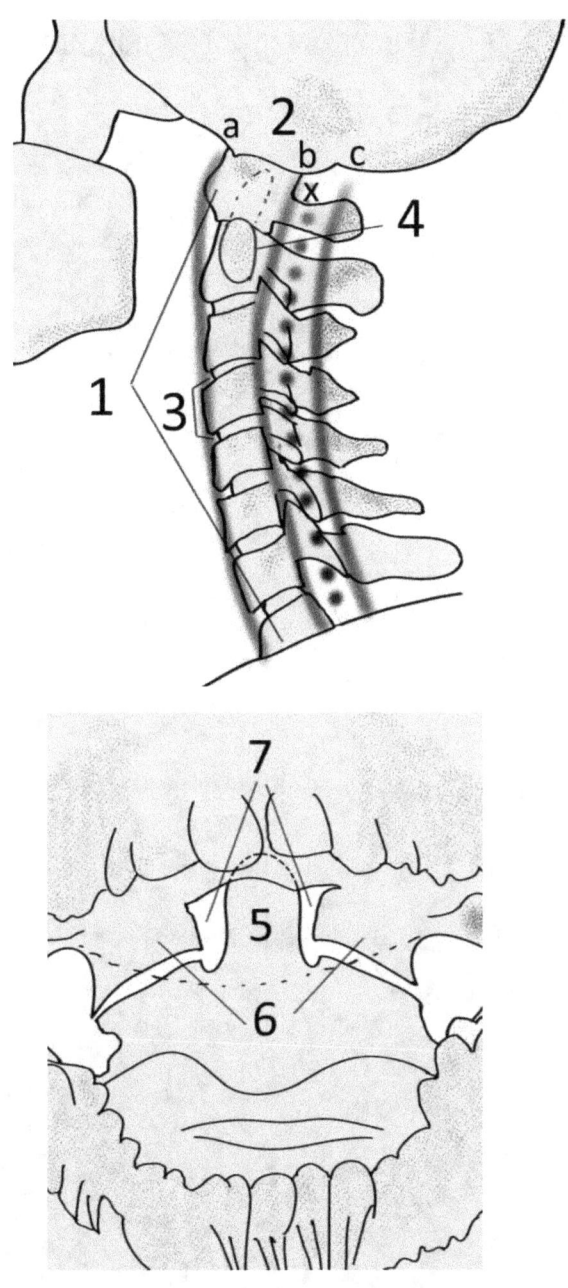

CHAPTER 2: GALLERY OF COMMON BONE FRACTURES

GROWTH PLATE (PHYSEAL) FRACTURES

SALTER–HARRIS VS AITKEN CLASSIFICATION.

Salter–Harris	Aitken	Description
I	0	fracture plane passes all the way through the growth plate, not involving bone
II	I	fracture passes across most of the growth plate and up through the metaphysis
III	II	fracture plane passes some distance along the growth plate and down through the epiphysis
IV	III	fracture plane passes directly through the metaphysis, growth plate and down through the epiphysis
V		crushing type injury does not displace the growth plate but damages it by direct compression

Mnemonic SALTR.
- ✓ Slipped fracture
- ✓ Above
- ✓ Lower
- ✓ Through or transverse or together
- ✓ Ruined or rammed

Salter–Harris vs Aitken classification

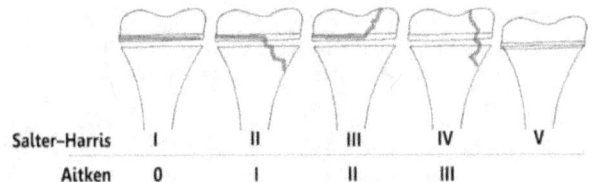

| Salter–Harris | I | II | III | IV | V |
| Aitken | 0 | I | II | III | |

FIBULA

DISTAL FIBULAR FRACTURE

A fracture of the distal third of the fibula (including the lateral Malleolus). It may affect also the distal tibiofibular syndesmosis and the deltoid ligament. This fracture is usually the result of an inversion injury with or without rotation.

WEBER CLASSIFICATION

	Weber A	Weber B	Weber C
Relation to the ankle joint	below the level of the ankle joint	At the level of the ankle joint	Above the level of the ankle joint
tibiofibular syndesmosis	intact	intact or only partially torn	disrupted
deltoid ligament	intact	intact or only partially torn	disrupted
Stability	usually stable	variable	unstable
management	conservative	variable	operative

> When examining a patient with an eversion ankle injury and clinical suspicion of medial malleolus fracture, always check the knee for proximal fibular fracture.

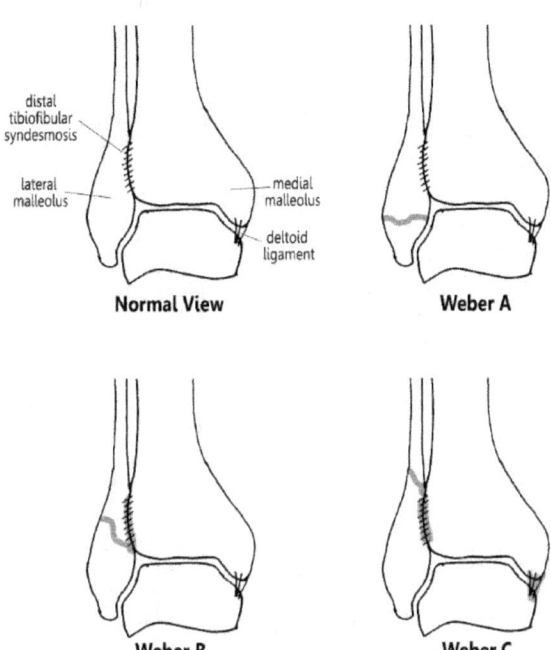

Weber classification of distal fibular fractures

Maisonneuve Fracture

A proximal spiral fibular is associated with distal tibiofibular syndesmosis rupture and the interosseous membrane. Usually associated with medial malleolus fracture or widening of the ankle joint.

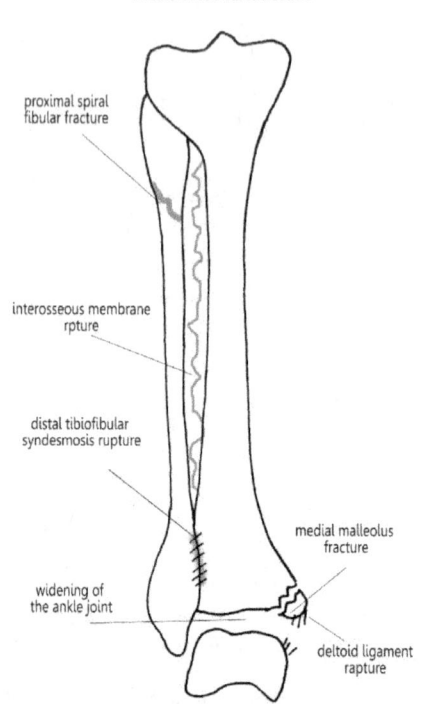

Maisonneuve fracture

proximal spiral fibular fracture

interosseous membrane rpture

distal tibiofibular syndesmosis rupture

medial malleolus fracture

widening of the ankle joint

deltoid ligament rapture

Le Fort
FRACTURE OF ANKLE

This is a vertical fracture of the antero-medial part of the distal fibula with avulsion of the anterior tibiofibular ligament

Bosworth fracture

This is a rare fracture of the distal fibula with an associated fixed posterior dislocation of the proximal fibular fragment which becomes trapped behind the posterior tibial tubercle.

POTT'S FRACTURE

Distal fibular fracture above the syndesmosis which remains intact. It is associated with deltoid ligament rupture and lateral subluxation of the talus.

Pott Fracture

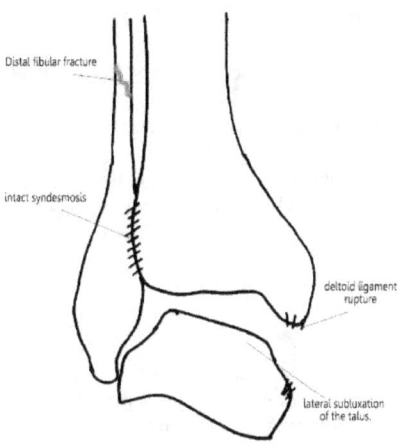

Distal fibular fracture

intact syndesmosis

deltoid ligament rupture

lateral subluxation of the talus.

Ottawa rules[1]

Ankle, foot and knee injuries are so common that a certain clinical criteria were developed to minimize the unnecessary X-Ray investigations. X-ray is only indicated in the following conditions.

OTTAWA ANKLE RULE
- Pain near one or both of the malleoli PLUS *at least one* of the following:

    o Bone tenderness at the posterior edge or tip of the lateral malleolus (the distal 6 cm).
    o Bone tenderness at the posterior edge or tip of the medial malleolus (the distal 6 cm).
    o Loss of the ability of weight-bearing of the injured foot. Inability to take 4 complete steps both immediately after the injury or at the time of the examination.

OTTAWA FOOT RULES

- Pain at midfoot zone (tarsal area) PLUS *at least one* of the following:
    o Bone tenderness at the base of the fifth metatarsal.
    o Bone tenderness at the navicular bone.
    o Loss of the ability of weight-bearing of the injured foot. Inability to take 4 complete steps both immediately after the injury or at the time of the examination.

THE OTTAWA KNEE RULE
- knee injury patients PLUS *at least one* of the following:

    o Age 55 or older
    o Isolated tenderness of the patella
    o Tenderness of the head of the fibula
    o Cannot flex to 90 degrees
    o Loss of the ability of weight-bearing of the injured foot. Inability to take 4 complete steps both immediately after the injury or at the time of the examination.

---

[1] http://www.theottawarules.ca

In Patients who don't meet these criteria, it is wise to advice RICE management plan with follow up in 5 to 7 days if the symptoms persisted.

RICE management plan:

Rest, Ice, Compression and Elevation.

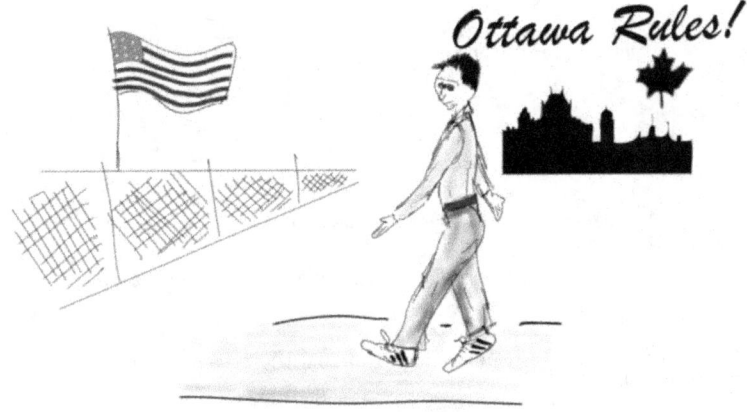

Canadian health system sucks, I am going back!

TIBIA

TIBIAL PLATEAU FRACTURE

SCHATZKER CLASSIFICATION

Type	Description
I	Wedge-shaped splitting fracture of the lateral tibial plateau.
II	Splitting and depression of the lateral tibial plateau; (type I fracture with a depressed component)
III	Pure depression of the lateral tibial plateau
IV	Medial tibial plateau fracture with a split or depressed component
V	Wedge-shaped splitting fracture of both lateral and medial tibial plateau
VI	transverse tibial metadiaphyseal fracture, along with any type of tibial plateau fracture (metaphyseal-diaphyseal discontinuity)

Type II is by far the most common tibial plateau fracture (75% of cases). In the second place is the Type IV (20% of cases).

Schatzker classification of tibial plateau fractures

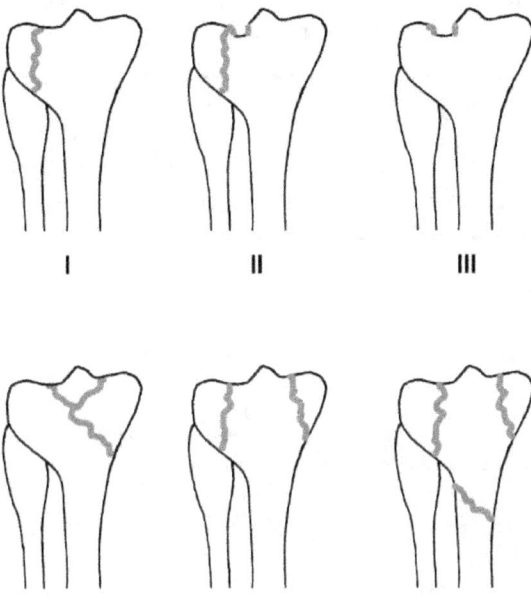

HOHL AND MOORE CLASSIFICATION OF PROXIMAL TIBIA FRACTURE-DISLOCATIONS

This classification is useful in fractures that couldn't be classified according to Schatzker classification or fractures associated with knee instability.

Type	Description
Type I	Coronal split fracture
Type II	Entire condylar fracture
Type III	Rim avulsion fracture of lateral plateau
Type IV	Rim compression fracture
Type V	Four-part fracture

BUMPER FRACTURE

A bumper fracture is a fracture of the lateral tibial plateau caused by a forced valgus applied to the knee. This causes the lateral part of the distal femur to compress the tibial plateau causing the fracture. Schatzker Type II.

> The classic mechanism of injury is when a car bumper hits the knee laterally with foot is held stable on the ground (weight-bearing limb).

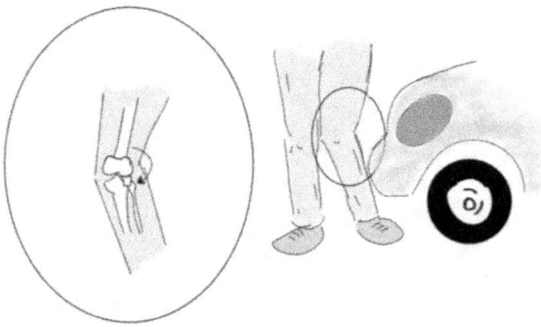

TIBIA SHAFT FRACTURE

This is a fracture of the proximal third of the tibia. It is usually associated with soft tissue injury or open wounds.

> Tibia shaft fracture is the most commonly fractured long bone in the body

OESTERN AND TSCHERNE CLASSIFICATION OF CLOSED FRACTUER SOFT TISSUE INJURY

Grade	Description
0	Injuries from indirect forces with negligible soft-tissue damage
I	Superficial contusion/abrasion, simple fractures
II	Deep abrasions, muscle/skin contusion, direct trauma, impending compartment syndrome
III	Excessive skin contusion, crushed skin or destruction of muscle, subcutaneous degloving, acute compartment syndrome, and rupture of major blood vessel or nerve

GUSTILO-ANDERSON CLASSIFICATION OF OPEN TIBIA FRACTURES

Type	Description
I	Limited periosteal stripping, clean wound < 1 cm
II	Mild to moderate periosteal stripping, wound >1 cm in length
IIIA	Significant soft tissue injury (often evidenced by a segmental fracture or comminution), significant periosteal stripping, wound usually >5cm in length, no flap required
IIIB	Significant periosteal stripping and soft tissue injury, flap required due to inadequate soft tissue coverage.
IIIC	Significant soft tissue injury (often evidenced by a segmental fracture or comminution), vascular injury requiring repair to maintain limb viability

Segond fracture

The Segond fracture is a type of avulsion fracture (soft tissue structures tearing off bits of their bony attachment) of the lateral tibial condyle of the knee, immediately beyond the surface which articulates with the femur.

Gosselin fracture

The Gosselin fracture is a V-shaped fracture of the distal tibia which extends into the ankle joint and fractures the tibial plafond into anterior and posterior fragments

Toddler's fracture

Toddler's fractures or childhood accidental spiral tibial (CAST) fractures are bone fractures of the distal part of the tibia in toddlers (aged 9 months-3 years). The fracture is usually found in the distal two thirds. It occurs after low-energy trauma, sometimes with a rotational component.

Pilon fracture Plafond fracture

This is a fracture of the distal part of the tibia, involving its articular surface at the ankle joint. Pilon fractures are caused by rotational or axial forces, mostly as a result of falls from a height or motor vehicle accidents.

The Ruedi-Allgower classification is a system of categorizing pilon fractures of the distal tibia.

Type	Description
I	*Non-displaced*
II	*Displaced but not comminuted*
III	*Comminuted articular surface*

Tillaux fracture

A Tillaux fracture is an epiphyseal fracture (Salter–Harris type III or Aitken II) through the anterolateral aspect of the distal tibial epiphysis. It occurs in adolescents between the ages of 12 and 15. In this age the medial epiphysis is already closed before the lateral epiphysis.

COMBINED TIBIA AND FIBULA FRACTURES

TRIMALLEOLAR FRACTURE

This ankle fracture is composed of 3 components: medial malleolus fracture, lateral malleolus fracture and posterior malleolus fracture. The posterior malleolus is a famous misnomer of the posterior part of the tibia, also known as Volkmann's triangle.

BIMALLEOLAR FRACTURE

This is an ankle fracture of both medial and lateral malleoli.

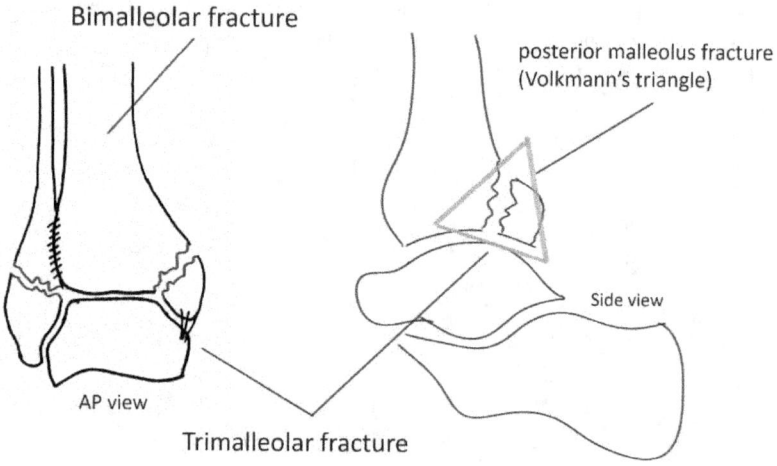

Bimalleolar fracture

posterior malleolus fracture
(Volkmann's triangle)

Side view

AP view

Trimalleolar fracture

FEMUR

FEMUR HEAD FRACTURES

PIPKIN CLASSIFICATION

The Pipkin is a system of categorizing femoral head fractures based on the fracture pattern.

Type	Description
I	Fracture below the fovea; not involving weight-bearing surface of the head
II	Fracture above the fovea; involving weight-bearing surface of the head
III	Type I or II fracture with associated femoral neck fracture
IV	Type I or II fracture with associated acetabulum fracture

Type III is associated with significantly increased risk of femoral head avascular necrosis.

Pipkin classification

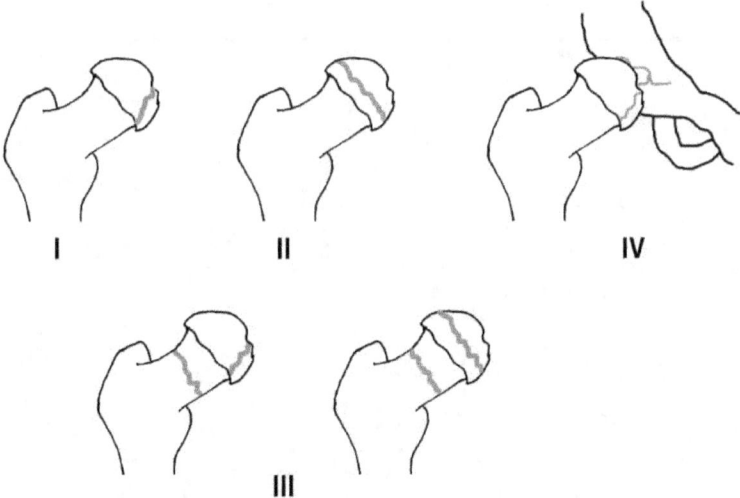

I   II   IV

III

Femur neck fractures

Garden Classification

This classification is based on AP radiographs only.

Type	Description
I	*Incomplete fracture or valgus impacted*
II	*Complete but non-displaced fracture*
III	*Complete, partially displaced fracture*
IV	*Complete, fully displaced fracture*

Simplified Version	
Non-displaced	*Includes Garden I and II*
Displaced	*Includes Garden IIII and IV*

Garden Classification

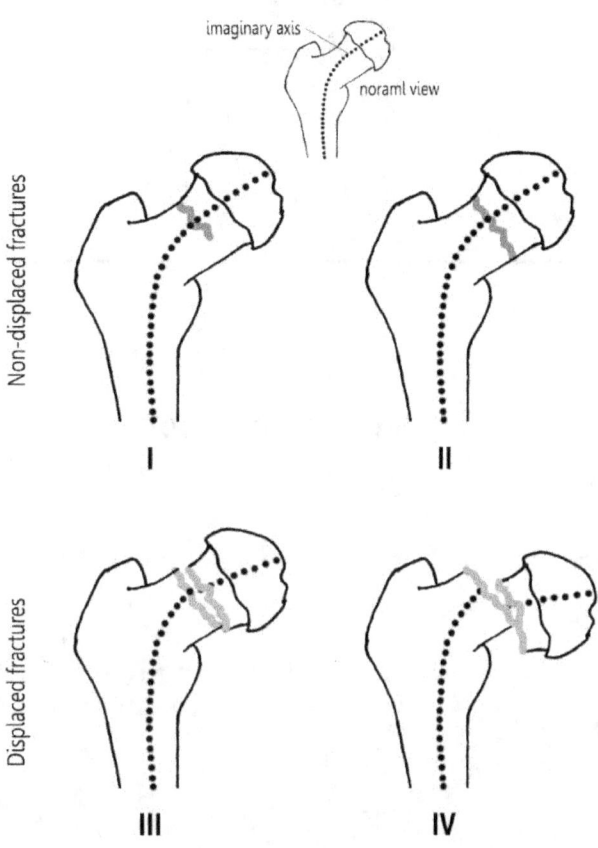

PAUWELS CLASSIFICATION

Based on vertical orientation of fracture line.

Type	Description
I	< 30 degree from horizontal
II	30 to 50 degree from horizontal
III	> 50 degree from horizontal (most unstable with highest risk of nonunion and AVN)

Pauwels Classification

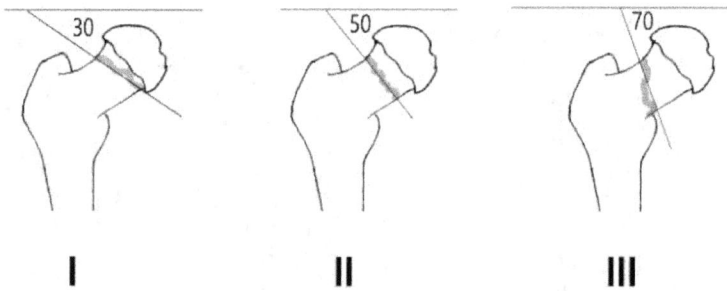

I   II   III

INTERTROCHANTERIC FRACTURES
EVANS-JENSEN CLASSIFICATION

Type	Description
IA	2-part non-displaced
IB	2-part displaced
IIA	3-part fracture with separate greater trochanter fragment
IIB	3-part fracture with separate lesser trochanter fragment
III	4-part fracture

MANAGEMENT OPTIONS OF PROXIMAL FEMUR FRACTURES[2]:

Some selected cases of Pauwels I fractures can be treated conservatively, otherwise surgical treatment is always recommended.

Timing of surgery: within 24 hours of admission except in unstable patients or patients under oral anticoagulant therapy.

FEMUR NECK FRACTURES
In patients with a displaced intracapsular hip fracture perform replacement arthroplasty (total hip replacement) if the patient:
- ✓ were able to walk independently out of doors with no more than the use of a stick, and
- ✓ are not cognitively impaired, and
- ✓ are medically fit for anaesthesia and the procedure.

Otherwise perform a hemiarthroplasty.

INTERTROCHANTERIC OR SUBTROCHANTERIC FRACTURES

In patients with trochanteric fractures above or including the lesser trochanter perform fixation with a sliding hip screw in preference to an intramedullary nail.

In patients with subtrochanteric fracture use an intramedullary nail.

---

[2] Hip fracture: management, Clinical guideline [CG124] – NICE guidelines. Published date: June 2011 Last updated: May 2017

Femur shaft fractures

Winquist and Hansen Classification

Type	Description
0	No comminution
I	Insignificant amount of comminution
II	Greater than 50% cortical contact
III	Less than 50% cortical contact
IV	Segmental fracture with no contact between proximal and distal fragment

Winquist and Hansen Classification

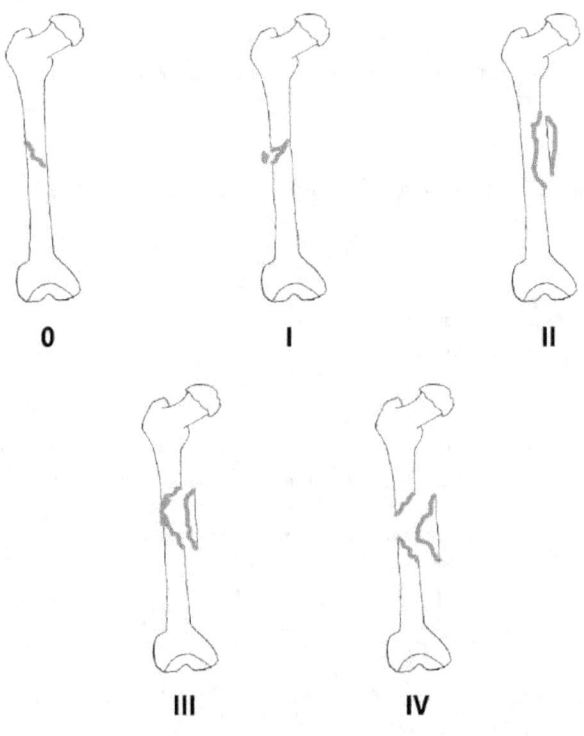

0 I II

III IV

PERIPROSTHETIC FRACTURE

VANCOUVER CLASSIFICATION

Type	Subtype	Description
A	A L	*Lesser trochanter*
	A G	*Greater trochanter*
B	B1	*Well-fixed prosthesis*
	B2	*Prosthesis loose*
	B3	*Prosthesis loose with poor bone stock*
C		*Fracture well below tip of the prosthesis*

Vancouver classification

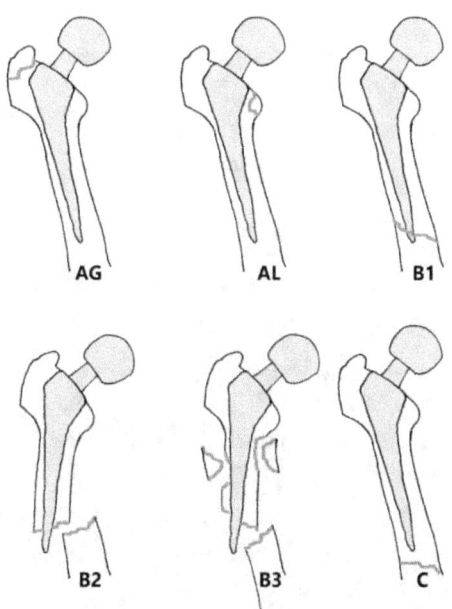

FOOT FRACTURE

LISFRANC FRACTURE

This is a fracture of the metatarsal bones associated with dislocation from the tarsus.

JONES FRACTURE

This is a between the base and the shaft of the fifth metatarsal bone.

MARCH FRACTURE

This is a fracture of the distal third of one of the metatarsals occurring because of recurrent stress. (Fatigue or stress fracture)

Foot fractures

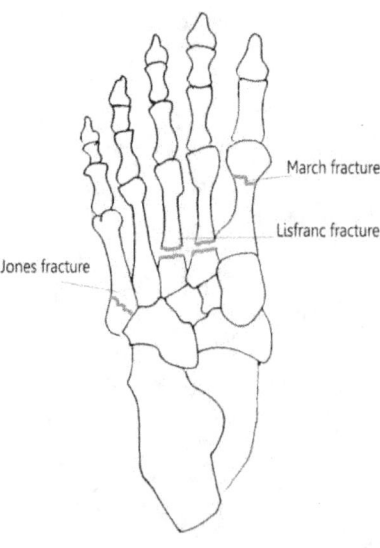

March fracture

Lisfranc fracture

Jones fracture

CALCANEAL FRACTURE

SANDERS CLASSIFICATION

Type	Description
I	Non-displaced posterior facet (regardless of number of fracture lines)
II	One fracture line in the posterior facet (two fragments)
III	Two fracture lines in the posterior facet (three fragments)
IV	Comminuted with more than three fracture lines in the posterior facet (four or more fragments)

PATELLA

TYPES OF PATELLAR FRACTURES

- Non-displaced
- Transverse
- Pole or sleeve (upper or lower)
- Vertical
- Marginal
- Osteochondral
- Comminuted (stellate)

> A strong clinical hint of the patella fracture is the loss of the ability of hip flexion while maintaining the knee extension.

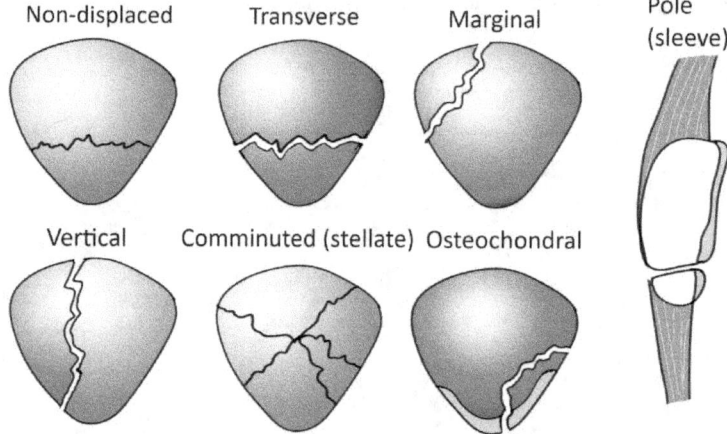

Non-displaced   Transverse   Marginal   Pole (sleeve)

Vertical   Comminuted (stellate)   Osteochondral

BIPARTITE PATELLA (TWO-PART PATELLA)

A congenital finding that may be mistaken for patella fracture. It is a patella with an unfused accessory ossification center at the superolateral aspect.

Features:

- ✓ It affects 8% of population.
- ✓ Characteristic superolateral position.
- ✓ Bilateral in 50% of cases.

PELVIC FRACTURE

THE YOUNG-BURGESS CLASSIFICATION

A system of categorizing pelvic fractures based on fracture pattern, allowing the judgment on the stability of the pelvic ring.

Type	Anterior Posterior Compression APC	Lateral Compression LC	Vertical Shear VS
I	Symphysis widening < 2.5 cm	Pubic ramus fracture and ipsilateral anterior sacral ala compression fracture	Posterior and superior directed force
II	Symphysis widening > 2.5 cm. Anterior SI joint diastasis. Disruption of sacrospinous and sacrotuberous ligaments	Rami fracture and ipsilateral posterior ilium fracture dislocation	
III	SI dislocation with associated vascular injury	Ipsilateral lateral compression and contralateral APC	

TILE CLASSIFICATION

Type	Subtype	Description
A: stable	A1	fracture not involving the ring (avulsion or iliac wing fracture)
	A2	stable or minimally displaced fracture of the ring
	A3	transverse sacral fracture
B: rotationally unstable, vertically stable	B1	open book fracture
	B2	lateral compression injury B2-1: with anterior ring rotation/displacement through ipsilateral rami B2-2-with anterior ring rotation/displacement through contralateral rami
	B3	bilateral
C: rotationally and vertically unstable	C1	unilateral C1-1: iliac fracture C1-2: sacroiliac fracture-dislocation C1-3: sacral fracture
	C2	bilateral with one side type B and one side type C
	C3	Also associated with acetabular fracture

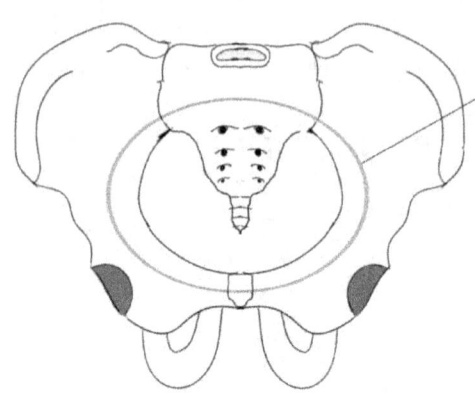

The stability of the pelvic fractures depends on the extent of damage of the pelvic ring.

Stable fracture: usually one undisplaced fracture of the pelvic.

Unstable fracture: more than one fracture of the pelvic ring at least one of then is displaced.

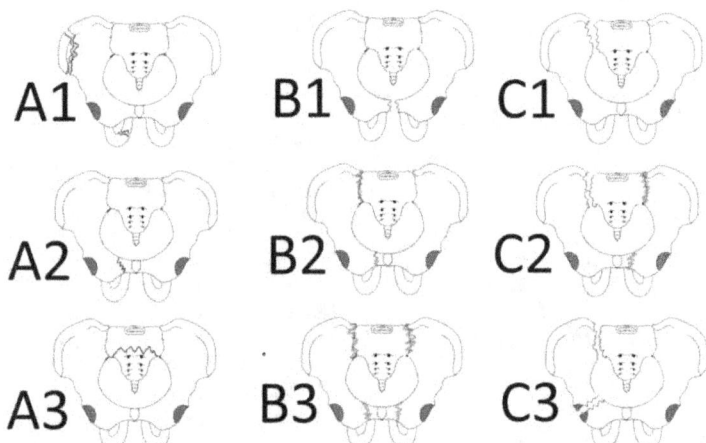

A1   B1   C1

A2   B2   C2

A3   B3   C3

OPEN BOOK FRACTURE

One specific kind of pelvic fracture is known as an 'open book' fracture. This is often the result from a heavy impact to the pubis, a common motorcycling accident injury.

DUVERNEY FRACTURE

Duverney fractures are isolated pelvic fractures involving only the iliac wing. They are caused by direct trauma and are generally stable fractures.

ACETABULAR FRACTURE

TILE'S CLASSIFICATION OF ACETABULAR FRACTURE

Type	Description
I	Simple fracture, anterior or posterior wall column
II	Transverse fracture
III	T - Type fracture involving two columns
IV	Both columns fractures, floating acetabulum

Shoulder Fracture

Middle Third Clavicle Fracture

Neer's Classification

Type	Description	Treatment
Non-displaced	Less than 100% displacement	conservative treatment
Displaced	Greater than 100% displacement Nonunion rate of 4.5%	operative treatment

Lateral third Clavicle Fractures

Neer's Classification

Type	Description
I	A minimally displaced fracture lateral to coracoclavicular ligaments with intact conoid and trapezoid ligament Stable fracture – conservative treatment
IIA	A medially displaced fracture medial to coracoclavicular ligaments with intact conoid and trapezoid ligament Unstable fracture – operative treatment
IIB	Two fracture patterns, both show signficant medial claviclular dispalcement Fracture occurs between the coracoclavicular ligaments. Conoid ligament is torn but trapezoid ligament remains intact Fracture occurs lateral to coracoclavicular ligaments with torn conoid and trapezoid ligament Unstable fracture – operative treatment
III	A minimally displaced intra-articular fracture extending to the acromioclavicular joint with intact conoid and trapezoid ligament Stable fracture – conservative treatment
IV	A laterally displaced physeal fracture with intact conoid and trapezoid ligament Stable fracture – conservative treatment
V	A medially displaced comminuted fracture with intact conoid and trapezoid ligament Unstable fracture – operative treatment

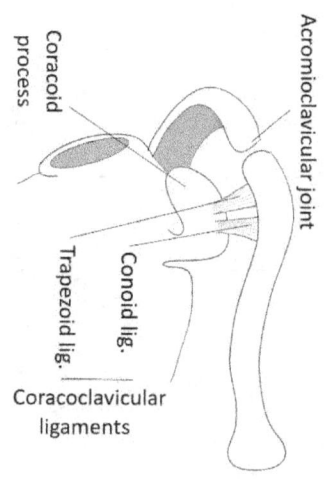

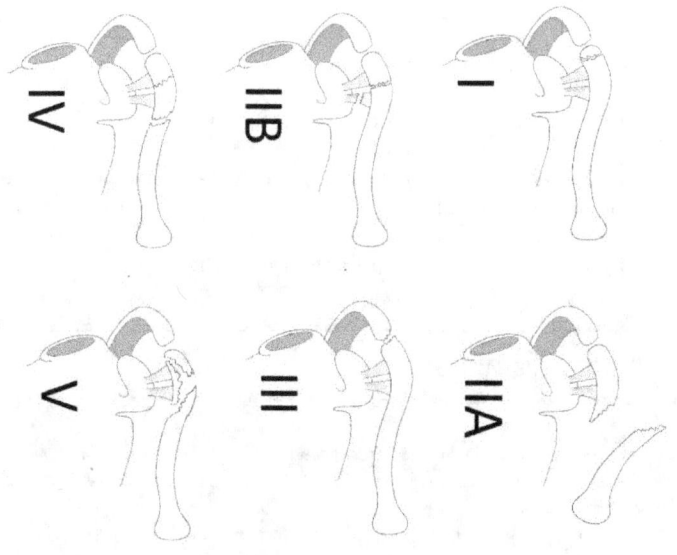

ACROMIOCLAVICULAR JOINT INJURY

TOSSY AND ROCKWOOD CLASSIFICATION

Tossy categories I to III are identical to Rockwood categories I to III. Furthermore Rockwood classification identify 3 more categories (IV to VI).

FURTHER CATEGORIES IF ROCKWOOD CLASSIFICATION

Type	I	II	III
Description	No radiological deformity	clavicle is slightly elevated	clavicle elevated above the superior border of kthe acromion
AC ligament	Mild sprain	Ruptured	Ruptured
CC ligament	Intact	Sprain	Ruptured
joint capsule	Intact	Ruptured	Ruptured
deltoid muscle	Intact	Minimally detached	Detached
trapezius muscle	Intact	Minimally detached	Detached

AC: acromioclavicular, CC: coracoclavicular.

Categories IV to VI are described as the category III with the following variations:

✓ **IV:** the clavicle is displaced posteriorly into the trapezius.

✓ **V:** the clavicle is markedly elevated where the coracoclavicular distance is more than double normal (i.e. >25 mm).

✓ **VI:** the clavicle is inferiorly displaced behind coracobrachialis and biceps tendon.

AC injury diagnosis

Clinically: tenderness of AC joint after a direct trauma. Piano key sign may be present.

X-Ray: the inferior borders of the lateral clavicular end and the acromion should be on the same level. If not, think of ligament injury. This can be assessed by measuring the following distances:

Acromioclavicular (AC) distance >8 mm: AC ligament rupture
Coracoclavicular (CC) distance >13 mm: CC ligament rupture

Humerus

Proximal fractures

Neer's Classification

Basic concepts of Neer's classification:

In this classification the proximal humeral end is divided into 4 parts: humeral head (or the articular surface), greater tuberosity, lesser tuberosity and humeral shaft.

The surgical neck separates the shaft form the tuberosities above while the anatomical neck separates the articular surface from the tuberosities below.

A fracture is regarded as displaced if the angulation is more than 45 degrees or the 2 fragments are displaced by more than 1cm.

Type	Description	Common pattern
One-part fracture	fracture lines involve 1 to 4 parts, none of them is displaced	Surgical neck
Two-part fracture	fracture lines involve 1 to 4 parts, one of them is displaced.	surgical neck (85%)
Three-part fracture	fracture lines involve 2 to 4 parts, two of them is displaced.	displaced greater tuberosity and shaft.
Four-part fracture	fracture lines involve 3 to 4 parts, three of them is displaced	Generally rare.

The terms one-part and two part etc. refers to the proximal humerus as a whole. In a one part fracture, in which nothing is displaced, the proximal humerus, despite being fractured, is considered as a ONE Part. On the other hand a two-part fractures means that one part is displaced (not only fractured) from the proximal humeral complex (the other Part).

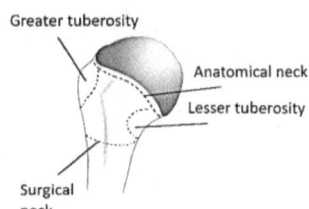

Greater tuberosity

Anatomical neck

Lesser tuberosity

Surgical neck

Neer I: minimally displaced fractures
Neer II: anatomical neck
Neer III: surgical neck
Neer IV: G. Tuberosity
Neer V: L. Tuberosity
Neer VI: Fracture-dislocation

	1 Part	2 Parts	3 Parts	4 Parts
I				
II				
III				
IV				
V				
VI	Proximal humerus fracture combined with anterior or posterior shoulder dislocation			

SUPRACONDYLAR FRACTURE

A supracondylar humerus fracture is a fracture of the distal humerus just above the elbow joint. This fracture is more common in children. There are 2 subtypes of this fracture according to the mechanism of injury: Extension Type (95% of cases - Hyperextension occurs during a fall onto an outstretched hand) and Flexion Type in only 5% of cases.

GARTLAND CLASSIFICATION OF EXTENSION SUPRACONDYLAR FRACTURE

Type	Description
I	non-displaced fractures
II	angulated fractures
III	Angulated with complete separation between the 2 fragments

> Neurovascular complications (The Pink and Pulseless hand) is relatively common in supracondylar fractures due to tear, spasm or entrapment of the brachial artery.

HOLSTEIN–LEWIS FRACTURE

This is a fracture of the distal third of the humerus resulting in entrapment of the radial nerve.

Ulna

Monteggia fracture

This is a fracture of the proximal third of the ulna with dislocation of the proximal head of the radius.

Hume fracture

The Hume fracture is an injury of the elbow comprising a fracture of the olecranon with an associated anterior dislocation of the radial head which occurs in children. It can be considered a variant of the Monteggia fracture.

Olecranon Fractures

Schatzker Classification

Type	Description
A	Simple transverse fracture
B	Impacted transverse fracture
C	Oblique fracture
D	Comminuted fracture
E	More distal fracture, extra-articular
F	Fracture-dislocation

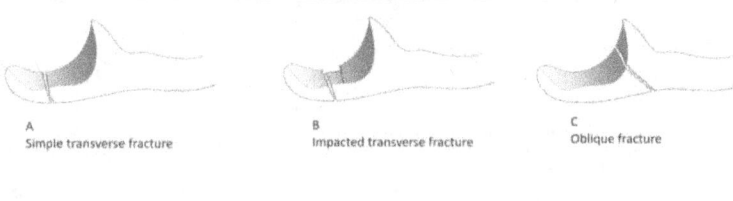

A
Simple transverse fracture

B
Impacted transverse fracture

C
Oblique fracture

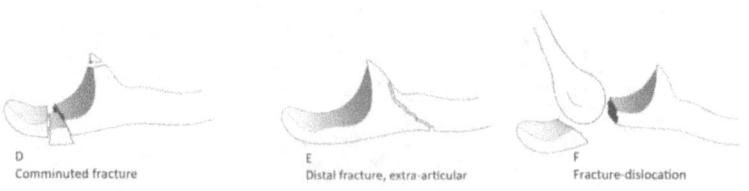

D
Comminuted fracture

E
Distal fracture, extra-articular

F
Fracture-dislocation

RADIUS

RADIAL HEAD FRACTURES

MASON CLASSIFICATION (MODIFIED BY HOTCHKISS AND BROBERG-MORREY)

Type	Description
I	Non-displaced or minimally displaced (<2mm), no mechanical block to rotation
II	Displaced >2mm or angulated, possible mechanical block to forearm rotation
III	Comminuted and displaced, mechanical block to motion
IV	Radial head fracture with associated elbow dislocation

Terrible Triad Injury of Elbow
✓ elbow dislocation (posterior)
✓ radial head or neck fracture
✓ coronoid fracture
One of the difficult fractures to manage due to persistent instability, stiffness and arthrosis.

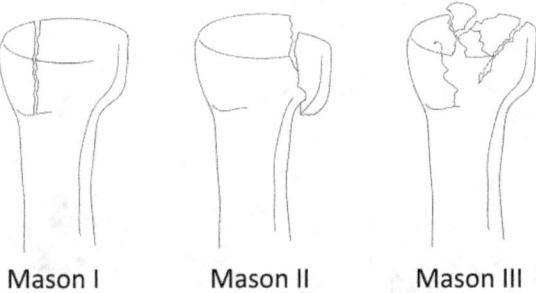

Mason I   Mason II   Mason III

ESSEX-LOPRESTI FRACTURE

This is a fracture of the radial head with concomitant dislocation of the distal radio-ulnar joint and disruption of the interosseous membrane.

GALEAZZI FRACTURE

The Galeazzi fracture is a fracture of the distal third of the radius with dislocation of the distal radioulnar joint.

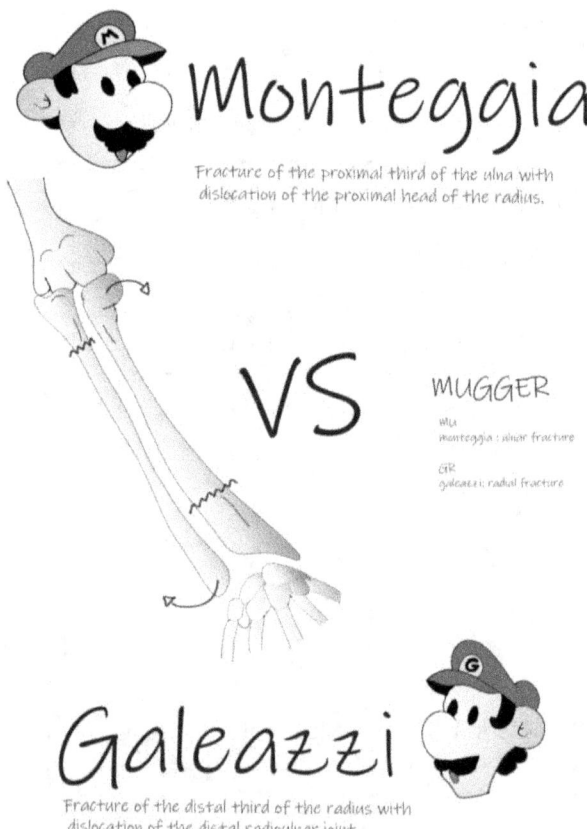

Monteggia

Fracture of the proximal third of the ulna with dislocation of the proximal head of the radius.

VS

MUGGER

MU
monteggia : ulnar fracture

GR
galeazzi : radial fracture

Galeazzi

Fracture of the distal third of the radius with dislocation of the distal radioulnar joint.

COLLE'S FRACTURE

This is the most common wrist fracture sustained in a FOOSH injury. It refers to a fracture of the distal radius with dorsal angulation and sometimes displacement of the distal fragment, producing a silver fork deformity. This term is used because the deformity resembles an upside-down dinner fork when the wrist is viewed laterally. This injury occurs most frequently in older women with osteoporosis

FRYKMAN CLASSIFICATION

Type	Ulna fracture absent	Ulna fracture present
Extra articular	I	II
Intra-articular involving radiocarpal joint	III	IV
Intra articular involving distal radio-ulnar joint	V	VI
Intra articular involving both radiocarpal & distal radioulnar joints	VII	VIII

SMITH'S FRACTURE

This is similar to a Colles fracture but the distal radius is volarly displaced. These fractures typically occur in younger patients and often are associated with other wrist injuries.

BARTON'S FRACTURE

This is a variant of Colles fracture in which the distal radius is sheared off, causing proximal migration of the distal fragment and dislocation of the radiocarpal joint. A Barton fracture requires immediate orthopedic referral for surgical repair

CHAUFFEUR FRACTURES FRACTURE

(also known as Hutchinson fractures or backfire fractures) these are intra-articular fractures of the radial styloid process. The radial styloid is within the fracture fragment, although the fragment can vary markedly in size

Hand

Scaphoid fracture

Fracture of the scaphoid bone is characterized by tenderness and swelling of the anatomical snuffbox. Complications may include nonunion of the fracture, avascular necrosis, and arthritis.

Mayo classification

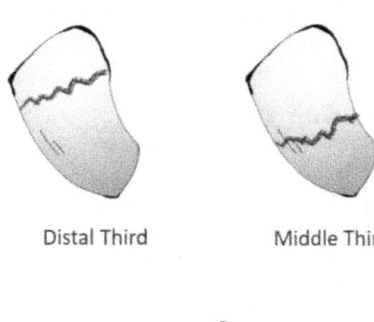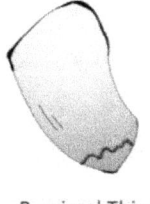

| Distal Third | Middle Third | Proximal Third |

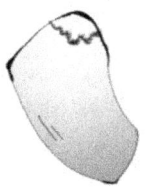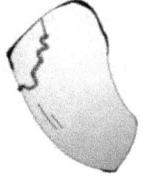

Distal Tubercle   Distal Articular Surface

Risk of avascular necrosis (AVN) depends on the location of the fracture.

✓ Fractures in the proximal 1/3 have a high incidence of AVN (~30%)

✓ Waist fractures in the middle 1/3 is the most frequent fracture site and has moderate risk of AVN.

✓ Fractures in the distal 1/3 are rarely complicated by AVN.

ROLANDO'S FRACTURE

The Rolando fracture is a comminuted intra-articular fracture through the base of the first metacarpal bone.

BENNETT'S FRACTURE

Bennett fracture is a fracture of the base of the first metacarpal bone which extends into the carpometacarpal joint. This intra-articular fracture is the most common type of fracture of the thumb, and is nearly always accompanied by some degree of subluxation or dislocation of the carpometacarpal joint.

BOXER'S FRACTURE

A boxer's fracture is the break of the 5th metacarpal bones of the hand near the knuckle.

GAMEKEEPER'S THUMB FRACTURE

(also known as skier's thumb) this is a type of injury to the ulnar collateral ligament (UCL) of the thumb. The UCL may be torn, damaged or in some cases avulsed from its insertion site into the proximal phalanx of the thumb in the vast majority (approximately 90%) of cases.

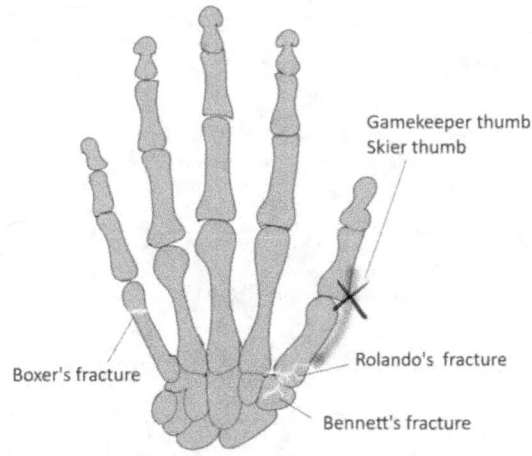

Gamekeeper thumb
Skier thumb

Boxer's fracture

Rolando's fracture

Bennett's fracture

Fall onto an outstretched hand (FOOSH)

A FOOSH is an acronym of a common mechanism of injury. A fall onto an outstretched hand can cause various fractures such as:

Common Fractures	Hint
Fracture of the clavicle	Look for deformity and tenderness of the clavicula
Fracture proximal humerus	More common in older patients. A similar injury in young people may result in shoulder dislocation.
Supracondylar fracture of the humerus	More in common children
Fracture of the head and neck of the radius	Adults: head of the radius, Children: neck of the radius
Monteggia fracture-dislocation	Probably with an element of rotation.
Galeazzi fracture-dislocation	
Colles' fracture	By far the most common type
Fracture of the scaphoid	Look for tenderness of the anatomical snuffbox
Bennetts fracture	fracture of the base of the first metacarpal bone which extends into the carpometacarpal joint
Gamekeeper's thumb fracture	Ulnar collateral ligament injury

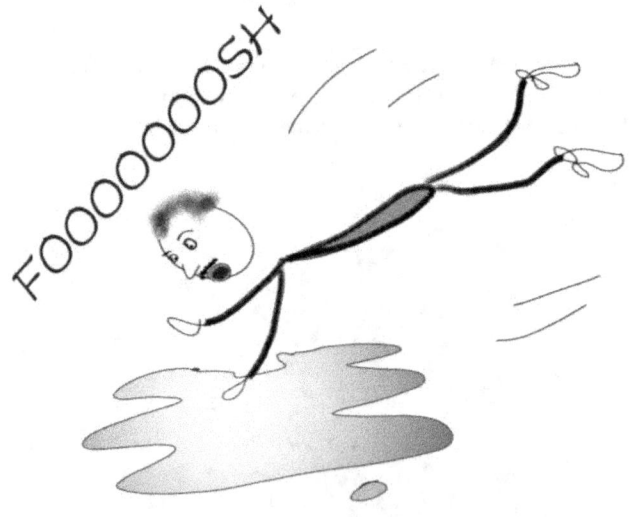

Vertebrae

Jefferson fracture

A Jefferson fracture is a bone fracture of the anterior and posterior arches of the C1 vertebra. Though it may also appear as a three- or two-part fracture. The fracture may result from an axial load on the back of the head or hyperextension of the neck (e.g. caused by diving), causing a posterior break, and may be accompanied by a break in other parts of the cervical spine.

Hangman's fracture

This is a fracture of both pedicles or pars interarticularis of the axis vertebra (C2)

Flexion teardrop fracture

A flexion teardrop fracture is a fracture of the anteroinferior aspect of a cervical vertebral body due to flexion of the spine along with vertical axial compression. A teardrop fracture is usually associated with a spinal cord injury, often a result of displacement of the posterior portion of the vertebral body into the spinal canal.

Clay-shoveler fracture

Clay-shoveler's fracture is a stable fracture through the spinous process of a vertebra occurring at any of the lower cervical or upper thoracic vertebrae, classically at C6 or C7.

FRACTURES OF THE ODONTOID PROCESS OF AXIS VERTEBRA (C2)

ANDERSON AND D'ALONZO CLASSIFICATION

Type I	rare fracture of the upper part of the odontoid peg above the level of the transverse band of the cruciform ligament usually considered stable
Type II	*most common* *fracture at the base of the odontoid* *below the level of the transverse band of the cruciform ligament* *unstable*
Type III	*fracture through the odontoid and into the lateral masses of C2* *relatively stable if not excessively displaced* *best prognosis for healing because of the larger surface area of the fracture*

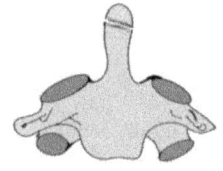 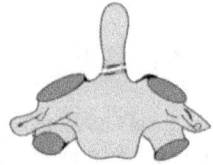 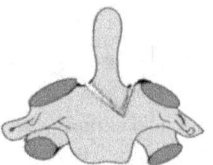

Type I   Type II   Type III

THORACOLUMBAR SPINAL FRACTURES

THREE COLUMN CONCEPT OF THORACOLUMBAR SPINAL FRACTURES
DENIS CLASSIFICATION

Denis divided the vertebral column into 3 vertical parallel columns based on biomechanical studies related to stability following traumatic injury. The fracture is considered unstable when it affects 2 adjacent columns. (i.e. anterior and middle column, middle and posterior column or the three columns).

Anterior column (AC)	Middle column (MC)	Posterior column (PC)
anterior longitudinal ligament (ALL) *anterior two-thirds of the vertebral body (VB)* *anterior two-thirds of the intervertebral disc (IVD)*	*posterior one-third of the vertebral body (VB)* *posterior one-third of the intervertebral disc (IVD)* *posterior longitudinal ligament (PLL)*	*everything posterior to the (PLL)* *pedicles (P)* *facet joints (FJ)* *ligamentum flavum (LF)* *Interspinous ligament (ISL)* *Supraspinous ligament (SSL)*

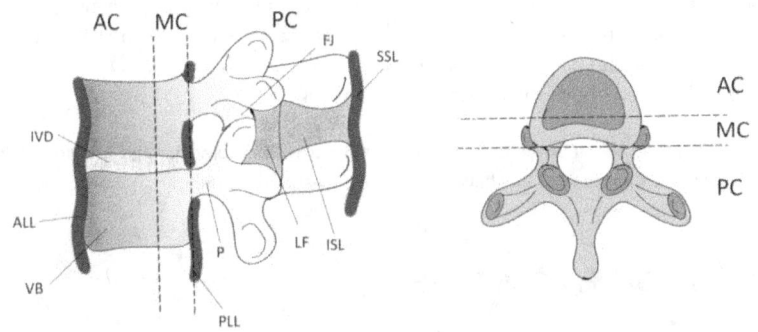

BURST FRACTURE

A burst fracture is a type of traumatic spinal injury in which a vertebra breaks from a high-energy axial load (e.g., traffic collisions or falls from a great height or high speed, and some kinds of seizures), with shards of vertebra penetrating surrounding tissues and sometimes the spinal canal. This an unstable fracture affecting the 3 columns.

COMPRESSION FRACTURE

A compression fracture is a collapse of a vertebra. It may be due to trauma or due to a weakening of the vertebra (compare with burst fracture). This weakening is seen in patients with osteoporosis or osteogenesis imperfecta, lytic lesions from metastatic or primary tumors, or infection. In healthy patients it is most often seen in individuals suffering extreme vertical shocks, such as ejecting from an ejection seat.

CHANCE FRACTURE

A Chance fracture is a flexion injury of the spine. It consists of a tension-failure injury to the anterior column of the vertebral body and a transverse fracture through the posterior elements of the vertebra and the posterior portion of the vertebral body. It is caused by violent forward flexion, causing distraction injury to the posterior elements.

The most common site at which Chance fractures occur is the thoracolumbar junction (T12-L2). Up to 50% of Chance fractures have associated intraabdominal injuries.

HOLDSWORTH FRACTURE

This is an unstable fracture dislocation of the thoraco lumbar junction of the spine. The injury comprises a fracture through a vertebral body, rupture of the posterior spinal ligaments and fractures of the facet joints

CHAPTER 3: AO/OTA FRACTURE AND DISLOCATION CLASSIFICATION

INTRODUCTION

This is a universal classification that applies numerical values to various types of bone fractures. This classification is a result of the collaborate work of the AO Foundation and the Orthopedic Trauma Association. This is particularly useful to create a precise and quick method of describing and documenting bone fractures. We will outline the general idea behind this classification, as well as a quick guide to use it with common fractures. For details and special cases, we would like to refer you to the Fracture and Dislocation Classification Compendium—2018, International Comprehensive Classification of Fractures and Dislocations Committee. J Orthop Trauma • Volume 32, Number 1 Supplement, January 2018.

BASICS OF AO/OTA FRACTURE CLASSIFICATION

AO/OTA Fracture and Dislocation Classification consists of several categories describing the bone fracture in detail. The main components are location and morphology. Location is described in 2 further subcategories Bone and location. Morphology is described in 3 to 5 categories according to the nature of the fractur itself. The first 3 categories (type, group and subgroup) are mandatory to describe the morphology. The 4th category (qualification) is an optional further description, while the last category (universal modifier) is a description of associated features like displacement or dislocation, or accompanying injuries like that of cartilages or ligaments.

Localization		Morphology				
Bone	location	Type	Group	Subgroup	Qualification	Universal modifier
1	1	A	1	.1	(a)	[1]
Numbers and upper-case letter separated by dots. It describes the affected bone.	Numbers 1-3. Describing which part of the bone is affected.	Upper-case letter A-C describing the general morphology of the fracture.	Number describing a specific feature of the type of the fracture.	Number after the dot describing a more detailed specific feature of the fracture.	Optional description of detailed features, lower-case letter within rounded brackets.	Number 1-14 with lower-case letter between square brackets describing a list of accompanying conditions.

STEP 1: LOCALIZATION-BONE

First order	Second order	Third order	
Thorax 16	Rips right 16.1.	Rips right from 1 to 12 16.1.1. to 16.1.12.	
	Rips left 16.2.	Rips left from 1 to 12 16.2.1. to 16.2.12.	
	Sternum 16.3.	Manubrium 16.3.1. Body 16.3.2. Xyphoid 16.3.3.	
Clavicula 15	Clavicula 15		
Scapula 14	Process 14A		
	Body 14B		
	Glenoid fossa 14F		
Arm 1	Humerus 1		
Forearm 2	Radius 2R		
	Ulna 2U		
Thigh 3	Femur 3	Patella 34	
Leg 4	Tibia 4	Medial malleolus 43	
	Fibula 4F	Lateral malleolus 44	
Spine 5	Cervical 51	C1 to C7 51.1. 51.7.	
	Thoracic 52	T1 to T12 52.1. to 52.12.	
	Lumbar 53	L1 to L5 53.1. to 53.5.	
	Sacral 54		
Pelvis 6	Pelvic ring 61		
	Acetabulum 62		
Hand 7	Capitate 73		
	Hamate 74		
	Scaphoid 72		
	Lunate 71		
	Trapezium 75		
	Other carpal bones 76		
	Metacarpals 77	1st to 5th metacarpals 77.1. to 77.5.	
	Phalanges 78	1st to 5th digit 78.1. to 78.5.	Proximal phalanx 78.5.1. Middle phalanx 78.5.2. Distal phalanx 78.5.3.
	Crushed, multiple fractures 79		

Foot 8	Talus 81		
	Calcaneus 82		
	Navicular 83		
	Cuboid 84		
	Cuneiforms 85	Medial 85.1. Middle 85.2. Lateral 85.3.	
	Metatarsals 87	1st to 5th metatarsal 87.1. to 87.5.	
	Phalanges 88	1st to 5th toe 88.1. to 88.5.	Proximal phalanx 88.5.1. Middle phalanx 88.5.2. Distal phalanx 88.5.3.
	Whole foot, crush, multiple fractures 89		
Skull and mandible 9			

STEP 2: LOCALIZATION-LOCATION

Each bone is further divided as following:

Proximal (or medial) part Equivalent to proximal metaphysis and epiphysis	1
Shaft Equivalent to diaphysis	2
Distal (or lateral) part Equivalent to distal metaphysis and epiphysis	3

Examples of fractur localization:
- ✓ Fractur neck Femur: 31
- ✓ Fractur Humerus shaft: 12
- ✓ Fractur lateral malleolus: 44
- ✓ Fractur of the base of the 5th metatarsal: 87.5.1
- ✓ Fractur of the shaft middle phalanx of the index finger: 78.2.2.2
- ✓ Fracture of 3 lumbar vertebra: 53.3
- ✓ Fractur of the posterior part of left 7th rib: 16.2.7.1

STEP 3: FRACTURE TYPE AND GROUP

ALGORITHM OF SHAFT OR DIAPHYSEAL FRACTURE LOCATION: 2

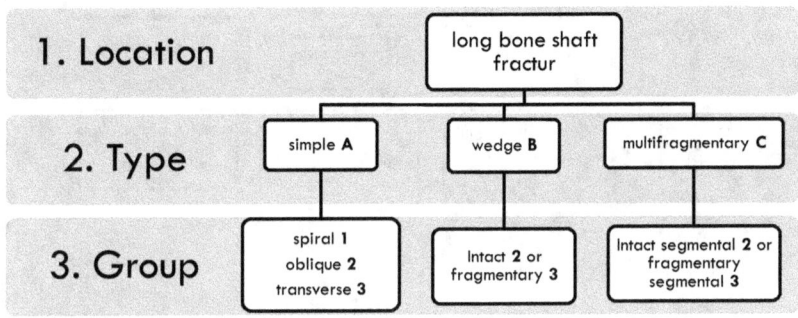

Examples

- ✓ Spiral simple fracture of the shaft of the humerus: 12A1
- ✓ Fragmentary wedge fracture of the 5th metacarpal shaft: 77.5.2B3

ALGORITHM OF END-SEGMENT OR EPIPHYSEAL FRACTURE LOCATION: 1 AND 3

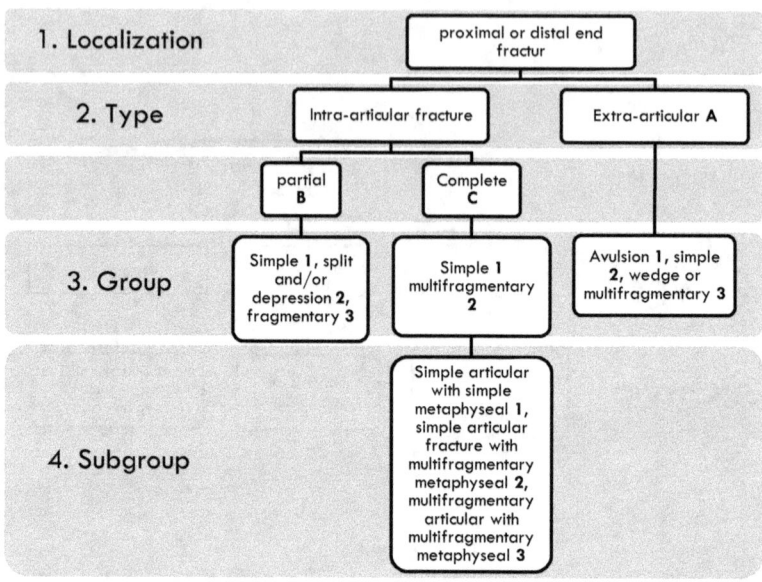

1. Localization — proximal or distal end fractur

2. Type — Intra-articular fracture | Extra-articular **A**

partial **B** | Complete **C**

3. Group
- Simple 1, split and/or depression 2, fragmentary 3
- Simple 1 multifragmentary 2
- Avulsion 1, simple 2, wedge or multifragmentary 3

4. Subgroup
- Simple articular with simple metaphyseal 1, simple articular fracture with multifragmentary metaphyseal 2, multifragmentary articular with multifragmentary metaphyseal 3

Examples
- ✓ Simple intraarticular fracture of the Head of the radius: 2R1B1
- ✓ Extraarticular multifragmentary distal radial fractur: 2R3A3

IMPORTANT EXCEPTIONS

Proximal Humeral und Femur fractures.

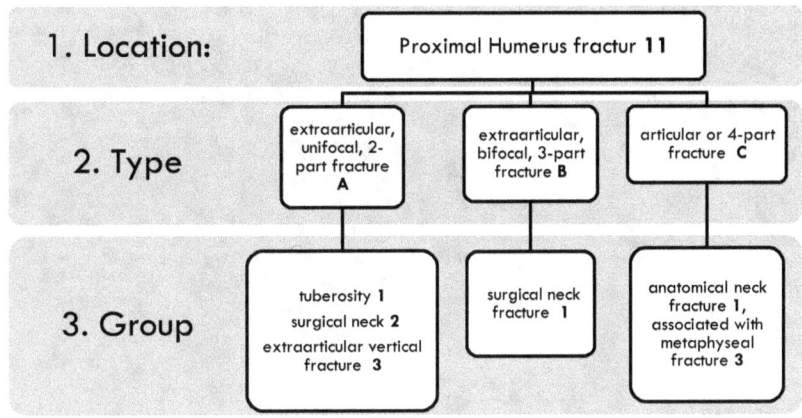

1. Location: Proximal Humerus fractur **11**

2. Type
- extraarticular, unifocal, 2-part fracture **A**
- extraarticular, bifocal, 3-part fracture **B**
- articular or 4-part fracture **C**

3. Group
- tuberosity **1**
  surgical neck **2**
  extraarticular vertical fracture **3**
- surgical neck fracture **1**
- anatomical neck fracture **1**, associated with metaphyseal fracture **3**

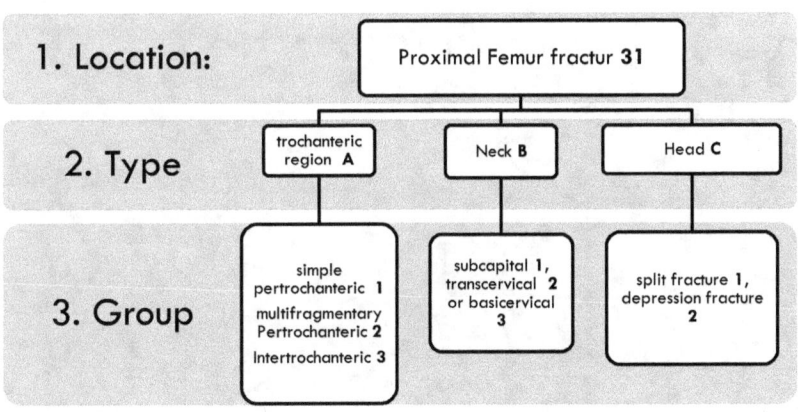

1. Location: Proximal Femur fractur **31**

2. Type
- trochanteric region **A**
- Neck **B**
- Head **C**

3. Group
- simple pertrochanteric **1**
  multifragmentary Pertrochanteric **2**
  Intertrochanteric **3**
- subcapital **1**, transcervical **2** or basicervical **3**
- split fracture **1**, depression fracture **2**

STEP 4: ADD UNIVERSAL MODIFIERS

1	Nondisplaced	
2	Displaced	
3	Impaction	3a: Articular 3b: Metaphyseal
4	No impaction	
5	Dislocation	5a: Anterior (volar, palmar, plantar) 5b: Posterior (dorsal) 5c: Medial (ulnar) 5d: Lateral (radial) 5e: Inferior 5f: Multidirectional
6	Subluxation/ligamentous instability	5a: Anterior (volar, palmar, plantar) 5b: Posterior (dorsal) 5c: Medial (ulnar) 5d: Lateral (radial) 5e: Inferior 5f: Multidirectional
7	Diaphyseal extension	
8	Articular cartilage injury	
9	Poor bone quality	
10	Replantation	
11	Amputation associated with a fracture	
12	Associated with a nonarthroplasty implant	
13	Spiral type fracture	
14	Bending type fracture	

Basics of AO/OTA Dislocation Classification

Site	Dislocation	Joint	Direction
1	0	A	[5a]
Numbers represents the distal bone of the dislocated joint.	0 is constant and represents dislocation.	Upper-case letter A-E describing the site of dislocation in joints formed of more than 2 bones.	Number 5 with lower-case letter a-e between square brackets describing the direction of dislocation.

Dislocation direction
5a: Anterior (volar, palmar, plantar)
5b: Posterior (dorsal)
5c: Medial (ulnar)
5d: Lateral (radial)
5e: Inferior
5f: Multidirectional

Examples of common dislocations

Remember to add the direction of the dislocation [5a-e] after the following code.

10 Shoulder	A glenohumeral
	B acromioclavicular
	C sternoclavicular
	D scapulothoracic
20 Elbow	A ulnohumeral with radiohumeral
	B radiohumeral
	C ulnohumeral
30 Hip joint	
40 Knee	A tibiofemoral
	B patellofemoral
	C tibiofibular proximal
70 Hand and Wrist	A distal radioulnar joint
	B radiocarpal joint
	C intercarpal joint
	D carpal-metacarpal joint
	E phalangeal joint
80 Foot and ankle	A syndesmosis
	B ankle joint (tibiotalar/talocrural)
	C hindfoot (subtalar joint)
	D midfoot
	E forefoot

Author's Biography

Mina Azer got his Master's degree in surgery in 2013. He has a great passion for science yielded in his current research and publications. Between 2004 and 2016 he shared in more than 70 different training delivered to more than 2000 trainees about various topics such as: reproductive health, surgical skills, and medical research. He worked at the Gastroenterology Surgical Center in Mansoura University, Egypt and at the Egyptian Liver Research Institute and Hospital. He is currently working at the Ubbo-Emmius Klinik in Norden, Germany.

Dear colleague,

Did we do a good job?
Is everything OK?
Is something missing?
Did we oversee something?
Perhaps a typo?
Is something outdated?

Your opinion is most appreciated. Please don't hesitate to contact us to share your insights to help us doing a better job in the next editions. Also like our Facebook page to stay tuned for updates, posters and cheat sheets.

All the best,

Yours,

Mina Azer
Email: meena_tharwat@yahoo.co.uk

Romany Azer
Email: r.azer@ ckq-gmbh.de

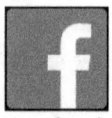

Facebook Page: A 2 Z in ER